Assessm

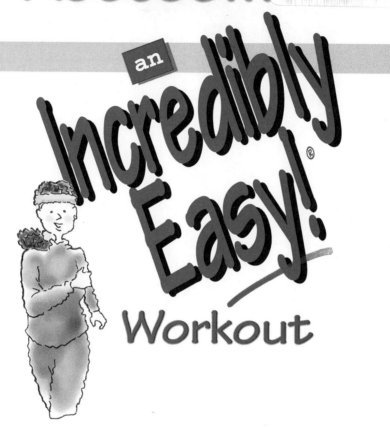

an

Incredibly Easy!®

Workout

Assessment

an Incredibly Easy! Workout

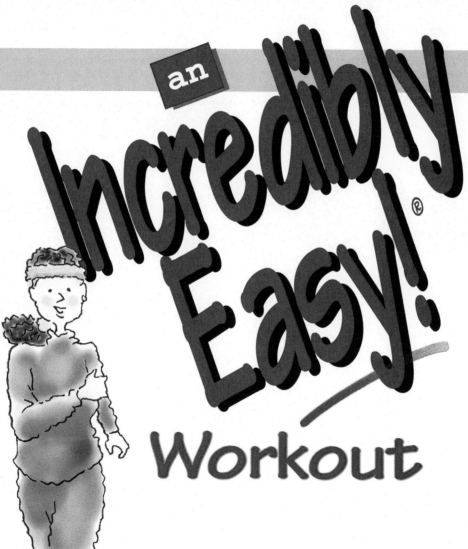

Workout

Wolters Kluwer | Lippincott Williams & Wilkins
Health

Philadelphia • Baltimore • New York • London
Buenos Aires • Hong Kong • Sydney • Tokyo

Staff

Executive Publisher
Judith A. Schilling McCann, RN, MSN

Editorial Director
David Moreau

Clinical Director
Joan M. Robinson, RN, MSN

Art Director
Mary Ludwicki

Clinical Project Manager
Kathryn Henry, RN, BSN

Editor
Diane Labus

Copy Editors
Kimberly Bilotta (supervisor), Pamela Wingrod

Designer
Lynn Foulk

Illustrator
Bot Roda

Digital Composition Services
Diane Paluba (manager), Joyce Rossi Biletz,
Donna S. Morris

Associate Manufacturing Manager
Beth J. Welsh

Editorial Assistants
Karen J. Kirk, Jeri O'Shea, Linda K. Ruhf

Workout regimen

1

Fundamentals

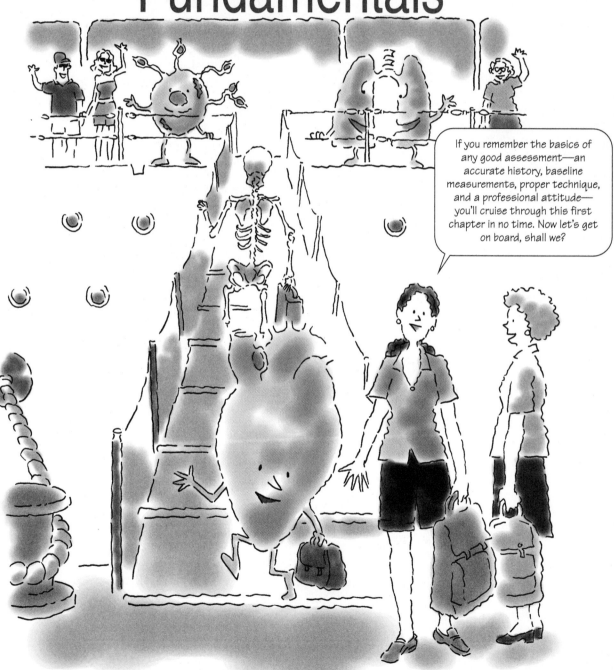

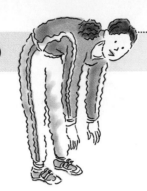

Fundamentals review

Health history

Obtaining assessment data

▪ Collect objective data (data that's obtained through observation and is verifiable).
▪ Collect subjective data (data that can be verified only by the patient).

Patient interview

▪ Select a quiet, private setting.
▪ Choose terms carefully and avoid using medical jargon.
▪ Use appropriate body language.
▪ Confirm patient statements to avoid misunderstanding.
▪ Use open-ended questions.

Effective communication

▪ Use silence effectively.
▪ Encourage responses.
▪ Use repetition and reflection to help clarify meaning.
▪ Use clarification to eliminate misunderstandings.

Components of a complete health history

▪ Biographic data, such as the patient's name, address, birth date, and emergency contact information
▪ Chief complaint
▪ Past and current health
▪ Health of the patient's family
▪ Psychosocial history (feelings about self, place in society, and relationships with others)
▪ Activities of daily living

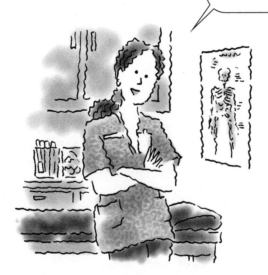

To make the most of your patient interview, create an environment in which the patient feels comfortable and use a variety of communication strategies throughout the history-taking process.

Physical assessment

Performing a physical assessment

- Introduce yourself and help alleviate the patient's anxiety.
- Explain the entire procedure, including expected duration.
- Briefly document essential information.

Body temperature

- Remember that normal body temperature ranges from 96.7° to 100.5° F (35.9° to 38.1° C).
- To convert from Celsius to Fahrenheit, multiply the Celsius temperature by 1.8 and add 32.
- To convert from Fahrenheit to Celsius, subtract 32 from the Fahrenheit temperature and divide by 1.8.

Pulse

- Remember that a normal pulse is between 60 and 100 beats/minute.
- To palpate a pulse, press the area over the artery using the pads of your index and middle fingers until you feel pulsations.
- Avoid using your thumb to assess pulse, and never palpate both carotid arteries at the same time.

Respirations

- Remember that 16 to 20 breaths/minute is normal.
- Assess respiratory rate while taking the pulse.
- Observe the number and rhythm of the breaths and the symmetry of the chest.
- Watch for the use of accessory muscles, wheezing, and stridor.

Physical assessment techniques

- Use drapes, exposing only the area being examined.
- Organize your approach: Start with the same body system; proceed in the same sequence.
- Perform inspection, palpation, percussion, and auscultation in that order for most body systems. However, when examining the abdomen, use inspection, auscultation, percussion, and palpation in that order.

Documenting findings

- Begin by documenting general information.
- Next, document information you obtained from your assessment. Record your findings by body system to organize the information.
- Use anatomic landmarks in your descriptions.

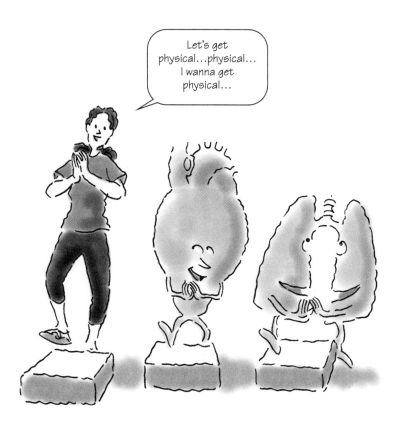

Let's get physical...physical... I wanna get physical...

Nutritional assessment

Evaluating nutritional status

■ Nutrition is the sum of the processes by which a living organism ingests, digests, absorbs, transports, uses, and excretes nutrients.

■ Nutrition includes adequate intake of proteins, fats, carbohydrates, water, vitamins, and minerals to ensure normal growth and function and maintain body tissues.

Obtaining a nutritional health history

■ Determine the chief complaint.

■ Obtain the previous medical history, family history, and list of current medications (including vitamins and herbal remedies).

■ Ask about the patient's routine activity level and eating habits.

Performing a nutritional physical assessment

■ Perform a general inspection.

■ Assess key body systems: skin, hair, and nails; eyes, nose, throat, and neck; cardiovascular system; respiratory system; and neuromuscular system.

■ Obtain anthropometric measurements: height, weight, and body mass index; when needed, midarm circumference, midarm muscle circumference, and skin-fold thickness.

Evaluating laboratory tests

■ Albumin: levels are decreased with protein deficiency, liver or renal disease, heart failure, surgery, infection, or cancer.

■ Hemoglobin: levels are decreased with iron deficiency anemia, overhydration, or excessive blood loss.

■ Hematocrit: is decreased in anemia; increased in dehydration.

■ Transferrin: levels reflect protein stores.

■ Nitrogen: intake and output should be equal.

■ Triglycerides: levels reflect lipid stores.

■ Cholesterol: levels are high with coronary artery disease.

Abnormal nutritional findings

■ Weight loss can occur with decreased food intake, decreased nutrient absorption, or increased metabolic requirements.

■ Weight gain occurs when ingested calories exceed body requirements for energy, causing increased adipose tissue storage.

■ Anorexia refers to a lack of appetite despite the physiologic need for food.

■ Muscle wasting occurs when muscle fibers lose bulk and length, causing a visible loss of muscle size and contour.

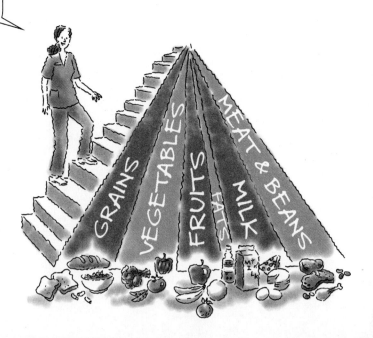

Mental health assessment

Obtaining a mental health history

▪ Establish a trusting, therapeutic relationship.
▪ Choose a quiet, private setting.
▪ Maintain a calm, nonthreatening tone of voice to encourage open communication.
▪ Determine the patient's chief complaint, using the patient's own words to document it.
▪ Discuss past psychiatric disturbances and previous psychiatric treatment, if any.
▪ Obtain the patient's demographic and socioeconomic data.
▪ Discuss his cultural and religious beliefs.
▪ Ask about a history of medical disorders; some conditions may adversely affect the patient's mental health.

Mental status checklist

▪ Appearance
▪ Demeanor and overall attitude
▪ Extraordinary behavior
▪ Inconsistencies between body language and mood
▪ Orientation to time, place, and person
▪ Confusion or disorientation
▪ Attention span
▪ Ability to recall events
▪ Intellectual function
▪ Speech characteristics that indicate altered thought processes
▪ Insight
▪ Coping or defense mechanisms
▪ Self-destructive behavior
▪ Psychological and mental status test results

Abnormal mental health findings

▪ Abnormal thought processes—derailment, flight of ideas, neologisms, confabulation, clanging, echolalia, incoherence
▪ Abnormal thought content—obsessions, compulsions, phobia, depersonalization, delusions, poverty of content
▪ Abnormal perceptions—illusions, hallucinations

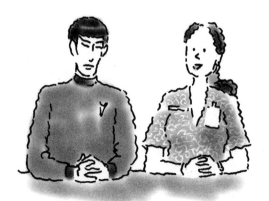

Yes, I guess it's logical to consider a mini-mental exam a type of superficial mind-meld workout. Shall we give it a go?

■ Batter's box

This is a fundamentally easy exercise. Fill in the blanks with the appropriate words and you'll be off to a great start.

Basic training

The patient assessment is composed of both an accurate _____ and a

detailed _____ . During the interview, you'll collect and record two

types of information: _____ data, which can't be verified by anyone

other than the patient, and _____ data, which can be obtained through

observation. You'll rely on your _____ skills and ask many specific

questions to determine the patient's _____ and to learn about his past

and current problems. Your physical assessment of the patient requires a systematic

approach and the use of four basic techniques (usually performed in this order):

_____ , _____ , _____ , and

_____ .

Special ops

Two areas that require special assessment are _____ and

_____ . A patient's nutritional health can influence his body's response

to _____ and _____ . Assessing a patient's appearance,

_____ , mood, thought processes and cognitive function,

_____ mechanisms, and potential for _____

can reveal a lot about his mental status.

Options

auscultation

behavior

chief complaint

communication

coping

illness

inspection

mental health

nutrition

objective

palpation

patient history

percussion

physical examination

self-destructive behavior

subjective

treatment

> When it comes to health assessment, don't be in a rush to swing at the first pitch. Take the time you need to do the job right, and you'll get a hit every time!

■■
■ Team up!

Write each assessment finding under its correct heading: subjective data or objective data.

Subjective data

_____

_____

_____

_____

_____

_____

_____

_____

_____

_____

_____

_____

_____

_____

Objective data

_____

_____

_____

_____

_____

_____

_____

_____

_____

_____

_____

_____

_____

_____

Findings
- Headache
- Blood pressure: 131/82 mm Hg
- Respirations: 22 breaths/minute
- Sore throat
- Cloudy urine
- Bleeding gums
- Tremors
- Tiredness
- Knee pain
- Dentures
- ECG results
- Weight loss of 15 lb
- Cough
- Eyeglasses
- Mottled skin
- Anxiety
- Difficulty walking
- Loss of taste
- Chest pain
- Temperature: 99.2° F

Two-minute time-out to review the assessment data play!

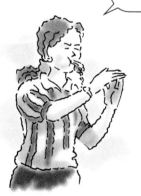

Cross-training

Complete this crossword puzzle, and you're sure to ace your next health history trivia competition.

Across

1. Head-to-_____ assessment

6. Indicator of disease

9. Of or relating to the heart

10. Data that can be verified only by patient

12. Drugs patient takes

13. Symptom commonly reported during patient history

14. System associated with breathing

16. Needed for vision

19. One who asks questions to gather information

20. Brother or sister

Down

2. Hormonal system

3. Normal, everyday activities (abbreviation)

4. Mnemonic device for exploring chief complaint

5. Uncontrolled body movement

7. Data obtained through observation

8. Bowel system

11. Type of personal information

14. Licensed nurse

15. Type of question that elicits yes-or-no response

17. Primary or main, as in _____ complaint

18. Nutritional intake

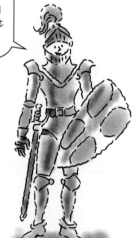

Cross-training back in the day...and this was with the light equipment!

Finish line

Identify the pulses pictured in this illustration.
(*Pulses shown:* brachial, popliteal, pedal, femoral, radial, carotid, and posterior tibial.)

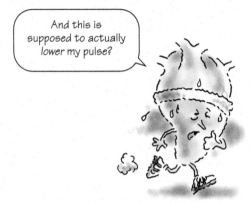

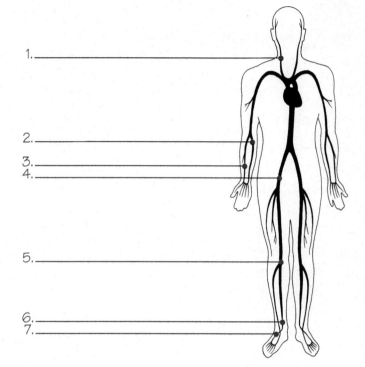

1. _____
2. _____
3. _____
4. _____
5. _____
6. _____
7. _____

Jumble gym

Unscramble the words below to learn important information about your patient's health problems. Then use the circled letters to answer the question.

Question: **What are you trying to pinpoint when taking a detailed patient history?**
(*Hint:* It's the main reason your patient is probably seeking health care.)

1. S U N B E N S M ◯ _ ◯ _ _ _ _ _

2. N O S E S H S T R F O H A R B E T
   _ _ ◯ _ _ _ _ _ _ _ _ _ _ _ _ _

3. R I N G C A M P ◯ _ _ _ ◯ _ _ _

4. I H A R S O L S _ _ _ _ ◯ _ _ _

5. N I T G H I C ◯ _ _ _ _ _ _

6. F L I D U T Y I C F G L O W S L A W I N
   _ _ ◯ _ _ ◯ _ _ _ _ . _ _ _ _ _ _ _ ◯ _ _

7. N I T C H T W I G _ _ _ ◯ _ _ _ _

8. H A S D E C H A E ◯◯ _ _ _ _ _ _

9. S H C E T A N I P _ _ _ _ _ _ _ ◯ _ _

Answer: _ _ _ _ _ _ _ _ _ _ _ _ _

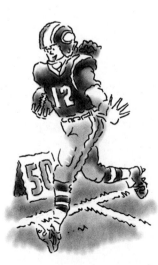

■ Mind sprints

Turn this closed question into an open-ended question to elicit more information from your patient. Time yourself, and see how many open-ended questions you can list in 5 minutes.

Closed question: **Do you have any pain?**

_____

_____

_____

_____

_____

_____

_____

_____

_____

_____

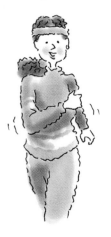

Keep an open mind about this exercise and then run with it!

■ You make the call

Identify the assessment techniques shown in the illustrations below.

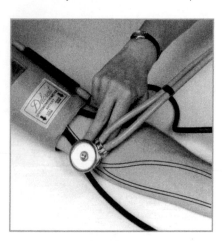

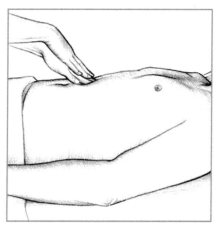

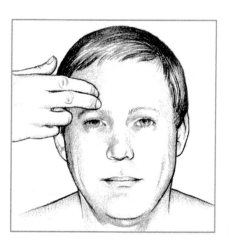

1. _____   2. _____   3. _____

■ Match point

Match the health history categories in column 1 with their definitions in column 2. (Some categories have more than one corresponding answer.)

Categories

1. Family history _____
2. Chief complaint _____
3. Biographic data _____
4. Activities of daily living _____
5. Medical history _____
6. Psychosocial history _____

Definitions

A. First information obtained in the health history

B. Includes detailed review of past and current problems

C. Normal, everyday routines

D. Pinpoints why patient is seeking health care

E. Identifies potential inherited risks

F. Includes revealing information about patient's feelings, relationships, and place in society

G. Personal identifying information, including name, address, telephone number, date of birth, nationality, and contact person

H. Includes information about parents and siblings and any known diseases

I. Includes information on diet, exercise, sleep, work, leisure, and use of alcohol, tobacco, and other drugs

J. Requires documenting patient's own words to avoid misinterpretation

Pep talk

"Life is often compared to a marathon, but I think it is more like being a sprinter; long stretches of hard work punctuated by brief moments in which we are given the opportunity to perform at our best.
—Michael Johnson"

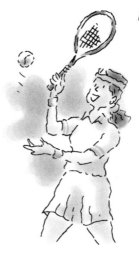

Something tells me I'd have a better chance against Venous System than Venus Williams.

■ Obstacle course

Can you identify five potential communication barriers interfering with the nurse's ability to conduct a thorough patient interview?

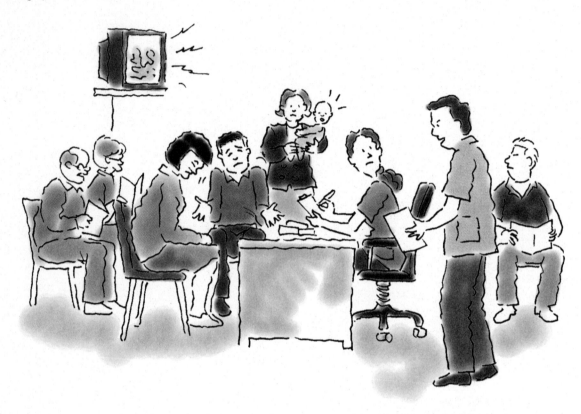

1. _____
2. _____
3. _____
4. _____
5. _____

■ Strikeout

Cross out the term that doesn't belong, and then identify the assessment step or technique characterized by the group of remaining words.

1. Body temperature, pulse, respirations, urine output, and blood pressure are part of a _____ _____ assessment.

2. Height, weight, head circumference, midarm circumference, skin-fold thickness, and visual acuity are considered _____ measurements.

3. Palpation, mental assessment, auscultation, inspection, and percussion are _____ _____ techniques.

4. Urinary, oral, rectal, axillary, and tympanic are common methods for assessing _____ .

5. Color, size, location, movement, texture, emotion, symmetry, odor, and sound are all assessed during the _____ _____ .

■ Match point

Match the vital sign in column 1 with the normal adult range in column 2. (Sorry, no units of measure in column 2— that would be way too easy!)

Vital sign

1. Temperature (Fahrenheit) _____
2. Pulse (beats/minute) _____
3. Systolic blood pressure (mm Hg) _____
4. Respirations (breaths/minute) _____
5. Diastolic blood pressure (mm Hg) _____
6. Weight (body mass index) _____

Normal adult range

A. 60 to 79
B. 60 to 100
C. 96.7 to 100.5
D. 16 to 20
E. 18.5 to 24.9
F. 100 to 119

■ Winner's circle

Circle the picture that shows the correct procedure for taking these anthropometric arm measurements.

Triceps skin-fold

1.
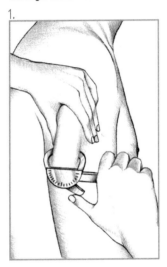

2.
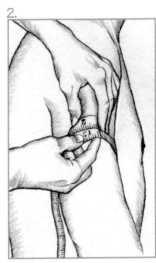

Midarm circumference

1.
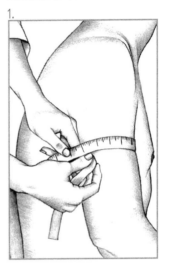

2.
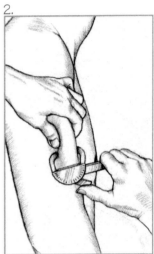

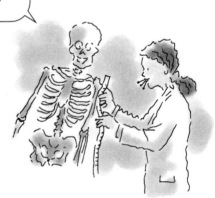

■ Batter's box

Fill in the blanks with the correct laboratory test from the box at right. Use each option only once.

1. Serum _____ level is used to assess protein levels in the body.

2. The carrier protein that transports iron is called _____ .

3. The main storage form of lipids, _____ are commonly measured with cholesterol.

4. _____ reflects the proportion of red blood cells in a whole blood sample.

5. A _____ balance test involves collecting all urine during a 24-hour period to determine the adequacy of a patient's protein intake.

6. A diet high in saturated fats raises _____ levels by stimulating lipid absorption.

7. _____ is the main component of red blood cells, which transport oxygen.

> **Options**
> albumin
> cholesterol
> hematocrit
> hemoglobin
> nitrogen
> transferrin
> triglycerides

How about loser treats the winner to a protein shake?

You're on!

■ Mind sprints

Nutritional problems can result from various factors, including physical conditions, drugs, diet, and sociocultural influences. Time yourself, and see how many factors you can list in 3 minutes.

Physical conditions	Drugs and diet	Sociocultural influences

■ Match point

Match the therapeutic communication technique in column 1 with what it aims to achieve in column 2.

Technique

1. Suggesting collaboration _____
2. Clarification _____
3. Rephrasing _____
4. Silence _____
5. Sharing impressions _____
6. Broad opening and general statements _____
7. Listening _____
8. Focusing _____

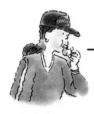

Sometimes self-communication can be very therapeutic.

Aim

A. Enables nurse to hear and analyze everything patient is saying and reveals patient's communication patterns

B. Gives patient the opportunity to explore pros and cons of a suggested approach

C. Attempts to describe patient's feelings, then seek corrective feedback to clarify misconceptions and gain better insight into patient's true feelings

D. Helps ensure that nurse understands and emphasizes important points in the patient's message

E. Initiate conversation and encourage patient to talk about any subject that comes to mind

F. Gives patient time to talk, think, and gain insight into problems

G. Demonstrates nurse's desire to better understand confusing or vague messages

H. Redirects patient's attention toward something specific and helps foster self-control

Coaching session
Conducting a health history interview

Choose a quiet, private setting for the assessment interview. Interruptions and distractions threaten confidentiality and interfere with effective listening. If you're meeting the patient for the first time, introduce yourself and explain the interview's purpose. Sit a comfortable distance from the patient and give him your undivided attention. If you're interviewing a patient with cognitive or memory losses, you may need to reorient him before beginning the interview.

During the interview, be professional but friendly and maintain eye contact. A calm, nonthreatening tone of voice encourages the patient to talk more openly. Avoid value judgments. Don't rush through the interview; building a trusting therapeutic relationship takes time.

■ Jumble gym

Unscramble the words below to identify commonly used coping mechanisms. Then use the circled letters to answer the question.

Question: What's key to all of these coping mechanisms used by patients?

1. ZAITAILORNATION _ _ _ _ _ Ⓞ _ _ _ _ _ _ _ _ _

2. LEADIN Ⓞ _ _ _ _ _

3. NASTYAF Ⓞ _ _ _ _ _ _

4. PETRJIOCNO _ _ _ _ Ⓞ _ _ _ _ _

5. RSINREPOSE _ _ _ _ Ⓞ _ _ _ _ _

6. GROSSINERE _ _ _ _ _ _ Ⓞ _ _ _

7. SPLICEDETANM _ _ _ _ _ _ _ _ _ Ⓞ _ _

Answer: _ _ _ _ _ _ _

> "Coping"...Geez, you guys are all amateurs! I've built my entire career around that one little word!

■ Hit or miss

Indicate whether the following statements are true or false.

_____ 1. A phobia is an irrational and disproportionate fear of an object or situation.

_____ 2. Hallucinations may be auditory, visual, tactile, somatic, or gustatory sensory perceptions that occur when no external stimuli are present.

_____ 3. The term that describes the feeling that one has become detached from the mind or body or has lost one's identity is an *illusion*.

_____ 4. Repetitive behaviors, or compulsions, result from attempts to alleviate depression.

_____ 5. Misinterpretations of external stimuli are called *illusions*.

■ Three-point conversion

Just when Nurse Joy thought she had heard it all! From the terms below, choose which abnormal thought process each patient is manifesting in the following illustrations.

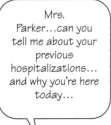

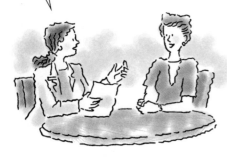

Mrs. Parker…can you tell me about your previous hospitalizations… and why you're here today…

…Parker…tell me about your previous hospitalizations …why you're here today…

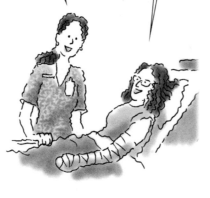

Oh, my! What happened to your arm?

I broke the yolk when I had a Coke. We all had a soak, and then I told a joke…

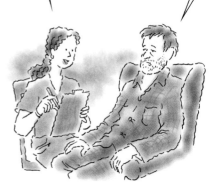

You were telling me about your childhood illnesses…

Oh, yes…when I was the young Prince of Denmark, we all had the bubonic plague and had to move to the summer cottage for an entire year. That's when I learned to speak nine different languages and got the German measles from my German nanny…

1. _____   2. _____   3. _____

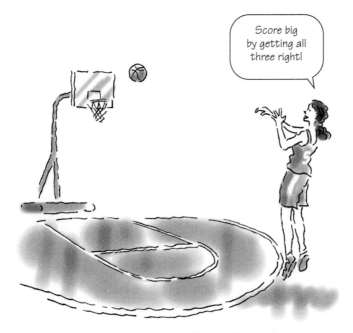

Score big by getting all three right!

Options

Clanging

Confabulation

Denial

Echolalia

Phobia

Rationalization

Repression

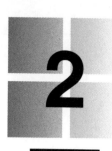

2

Skin, hair, and nails

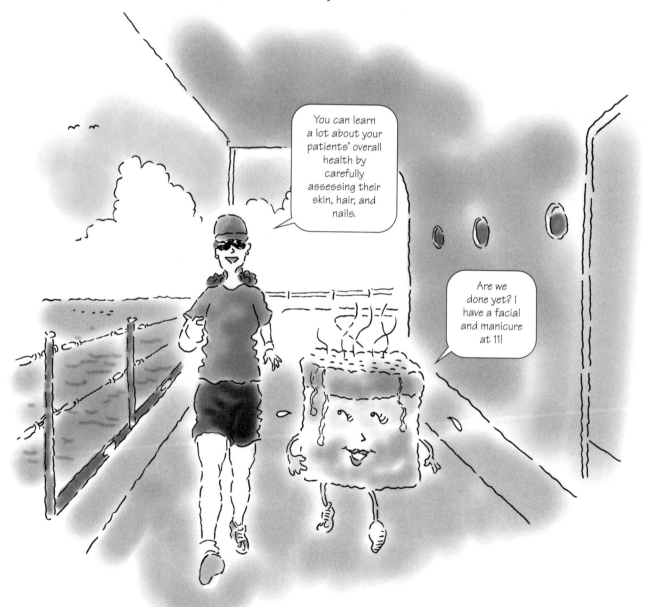

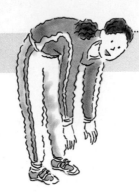

■ Warm-up

Skin, hair, and nails review

Health history

- Determine the patient's chief complaint.
- Ask about skin changes, lesions, and exposure to sun.
- Ask about a family history of allergies or skin cancer.
- Ask about hair loss or gain and sudden or gradual nail changes.
- Ask about signs and symptoms, such as discharge, fever, weight loss, and joint pain.
- Determine which medications the patient takes, including herbal preparations.

Skin

Structures

- Epidermis—thin outer layer composed of epithelial tissue
- Dermis—thick, deeper layer containing blood vessels, lymphatic vessels, nerves, hair follicles, and sweat and sebaceous glands
- Subcutaneous tissue—innermost layer

Functions

- Protects tissues
- Prevents water and electrolyte losses
- Senses temperature, pain, touch, and pressure
- Regulates body temperature
- Synthesizes vitamin D
- Promotes wound repair

Assessment

- Inspect and palpate the texture (should be smooth and intact).
- Observe for moisture content (should be dry with a minimal amount of perspiration).
- Palpate the skin for temperature, checking each side for localized temperature changes.
- Observe for skin lesions.

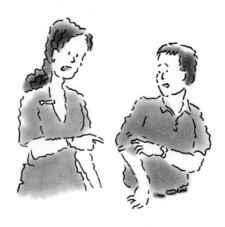

We've had a recent rash of rashes, Roger. (Bet you can't say that five times really fast!)

Lesion assessment

- Classify lesion as primary or secondary.
- Determine if it's solid or fluid-filled.
- Check borders to see if they're regular or irregular.
- Note lesion's color, pattern, location, and distribution.
- Measure lesion's diameter with a millimeter-centimeter ruler.
- Describe drainage, noting type, color, amount, and odor.

Abnormal findings

- Café-au-lait spots—flat, light brown, uniformly hyperpigmented macules or patches on skin surface
- Cherry angiomas—tiny, bright red, round papules that may become brown over time
- Papular rash—small, raised, circumscribed, and discolored (red to purple) lesions appearing in various configurations
- Port-wine hemangiomas—flat, purple marks usually present at birth; may appear on the face and upper body
- Pruritus —unpleasant itching sensation
- Purpuric lesions—petechiae (brown, pinpoint lesions); ecchymoses (bluish or purplish discolorations); hematomas (masses of accumulated blood)
- Telangiectases—permanently dilated, small blood vessels typically in a weblike pattern
- Urticaria—vascular skin reaction of transient pruritic wheals
- Vesicular rash—scattered or linear distribution of blisterlike lesions filled with clear, cloudy, or bloody fluid

Hair

- Formed from keratin
- Lies in hair follicle, receives nourishment from papilla, and is attached at base by arrector pili

Assessment

- Inspect and palpate hair over patient's entire body, noting distribution, quantity, texture, and color.
- Check for patterns of hair loss and growth.
- Inspect scalp for erythema, scaling, and encrustations.

Abnormal findings

- Alopecia—hair loss
- Hirsutism—excessive hairiness in women

Nails

Structures

- Nail root (or nail matrix)—site of nail growth
- Nail plate—visible, hardened layer covering fingertip
- Lunula—white, crescent-shaped area extending past cuticle

Assessment

- Examine nails for color, shape, thickness, and consistency.

Abnormal findings

- Beau's lines—transverse depressions extending to nail bed
- Clubbing—proximal end of nail elevates so the angle is greater than 180 degrees
- Koilonychia—thin, spoon-shaped nails with lateral edges that tilt upward
- Onycholysis—nail plate loosening with separation from nail bed
- Terry's nails—transverse bands of white covering nail

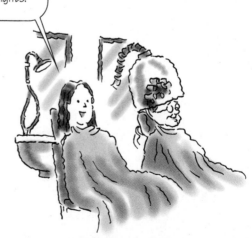

Remember that workouts—especially outdoor activities—can be especially drying to the skin and hair. Use plenty of sunscreen and moisturizer, and don't forget to condition those new highlights.

■ Batter's box

This exercise will test your knowledge of the integumentary system. Fill in the blanks with the appropriate words from the box. One word is used twice.

A big cover-up

_____ covers the body's internal structures and protects them from the outside
₁

world. The body's largest _____ , it has several important functions, including:
₂

■ protecting underlying _____ from trauma and bacteria
₃

■ preventing loss of _____ and _____ from the body
₄   ₅

■ sensing and regulating body _____
₆

■ promoting _____ repair.
₇

Skin has two layers, the _____ and the _____ , and an underlying
₈   ₉

layer of _____ tissue.
₁₀

The mane event

Hair is formed from _____ and produced by matrix cells in the dermal layer. Each
₁₁

hair lies in a hair _____ and receives nourishment from _____ .
₁₂   ₁₃

A hair bulb located at the end of the hair shaft contains _____ , which determine
₁₄

hair color.

A neonate's skin is covered with _____ , a fine, downy growth of hair that
₁₅

disappears several weeks after birth. _____ occurs in many people as a normal
₁₆

result of aging; in younger people, it's _____ determined.
₁₇

Pretty in pink

Nails are formed when epidermal cells are converted into hard plates of _____ .
₁₈

They're made up a nail root, nail plate, nail bed, lunula, nail folds, and _____ . With
₁₉

age, nail growth slows and nails become brittle and thin. Longitudinal _____ in the
₂₀

nail plate become more pronounced and make nails prone to splitting.

Options

balding

cuticle

dermis

electrolytes

epidermis

follicle

genetically

keratin

lanugo

melanocytes

organ

papilla

ridges

skin

subcutaneous

temperature

tissues

water

wound

■ Team up!

Write each skin structure under the skin layer in which it's found.

Epidermis

_____

_____

_____

_____

_____

Dermis

_____

_____

_____

_____

_____

Skin structures
- Apocrine (sebaceous) gland
- Blood vessel
- Eccrine (sweat) gland
- Hair follicle
- Lymphatic vessel
- Melanocyte
- Nerve
- Stratum corneum
- Stratum germinativum

Remember, one sign of a good workout is when those eccrine glands begin to kick in.

■ Jumble gym

Unscramble the words below to discover common characteristics associated with normal skin changes. Then use the circled letters to answer the question.

Question: **What condition would you expect in a patient with these skin characteristics?** (*Hint:* Unfortunately it's incurable and, for many, inevitable.)

1. RYD DAN KLYAF 〇_ _   _ _ _   _ 〇_ _

2. APEL CROOL _ _ _ _   _ 〇_ _ _

3. GENTNIT _ _ _ _ _ 〇

4. KNILWRING _ _ _ _ 〇_ _ _

5. CAPHMEEKLIRTN _ _ _ _ _ _ 〇_ _ _ _

Answer: _ _ _   _ _ _

Finish line

Label the major structures identified in this cross section of the skin.

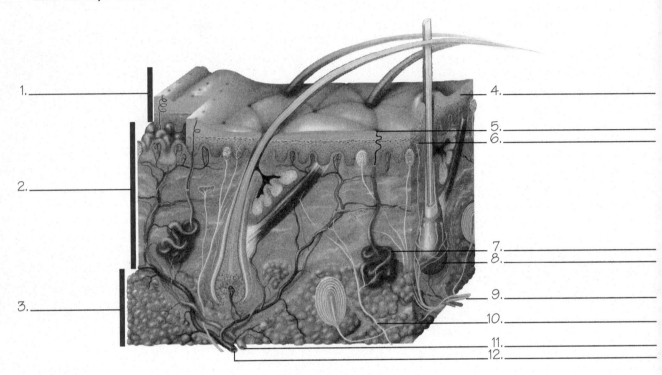

1. _____

2. _____

3. _____

4. _____

5. _____

6. _____

7. _____

8. _____

9. _____

10. _____

11. _____

12. _____

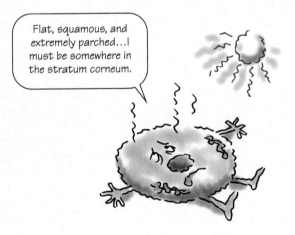

Flat, squamous, and extremely parched...I must be somewhere in the stratum corneum.

■■ ■Hit or miss

Indicate whether the following statements are true or false.

_____ 1. The stratum corneum is made up of cells that form in the basal layer and migrate to the skin's outer surface, where they survive for years.

_____ 2. Sebaceous glands are found primarily in the scalp, face, palms and soles, and genital region.

_____ 3. One of the most common complaints about skin is itching.

_____ 4. Rough, dry skin is common in patients with hypothyroidism, psoriasis, and excessive keratinization.

_____ 5. Irregularly shaped areas of deep blue discoloration that are a normal variation in Black and Asian children are known as port-wine stains.

_____ 6. Red lesions caused by vascular changes include hemangiomas, petechiae, ecchymoses, and purpura.

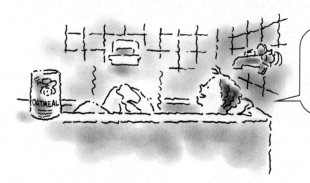

There's nothing like an oatmeal bath to soothe dry, itchy skin, especially after a hard workout.

■■ ■You make the call

Describe the assessment procedure illustrated below. Then tell how you would document the finding in your nurse's notes.

Procedure: _____

_____

Assessment finding: _____

_____

_____

_____

_____

_____

■■
■ Finish line

Label the parts of the hair shaft and glands shown in the illustration below.

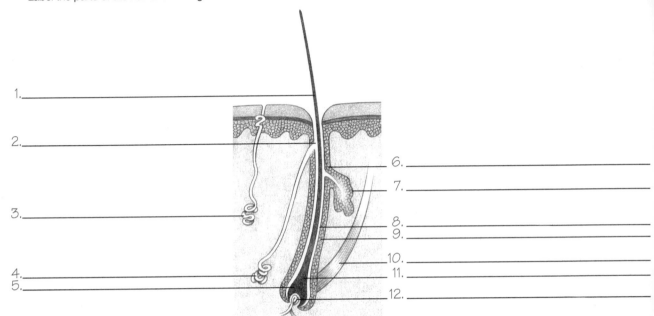

1. _____

2. _____

3. _____

4. _____
5. _____

6. _____

7. _____

8. _____
9. _____

10. _____
11. _____
12. _____

■■
■ Train your brain

Sound out each group of pictures and symbols to reveal the answer to this assessment-related question.

Question: **What equipment should you use if you suspect a patient has ringworm?**

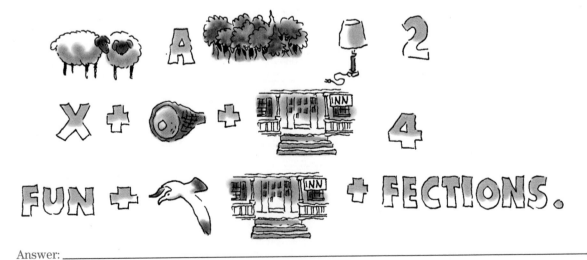

Answer: _____

■ Mind sprints

Go the distance by exploring a patient's chief complaint of "nail changes." Time yourself, and see how many nail assessment questions you can list in 5 minutes.

_____

_____

_____

_____

_____

_____

_____

_____

_____

_____

■ Gear up!

Choose which equipment and supplies you'll need to gather before performing a skin, hair, and nails assessment.

☐ Bulb syringe
☐ Tongue blade
☐ Clear ruler (with mm and cm markings)
☐ Penlight, flashlight
☐ Wood's lamp
☐ Speculum
☐ Scale

☐ Percussion hammer
☐ Stethoscope
☐ Magnifying glass
☐ Otoscope
☐ Thermometer
☐ Tuning fork
☐ Gloves

■ Match point

Match the skin assessment finding in column 1 with its general corresponding color variation in column 2. One color is used more than once,

Assessment finding

1. Mongolian spots _____
2. Erythema _____
3. Jaundice _____
4. Pallor _____
5. Cyanosis _____
6. Telangiectases _____
7. Carotenemia _____
8. Port-wine stain _____
9. Freckles _____
10. Butterfly rash _____

Color

A. Yellow

B. Red

C. Pink

D. Purple

E. Reddish-brown

F. Blue

G. Ash-white

H. Yellowish-orange

I. Tan to brown

In case you're wondering, I'm a natural red—with or without the workout.

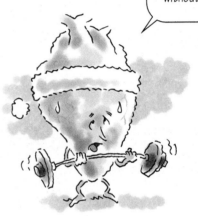

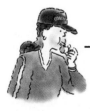

Coaching session

Detecting color variations in dark-skinned patients

When assessing a dark-skinned patient, keep in mind that color changes may vary depending on skin pigmentation. You'll need to look for other indicators to guide your assessment.

Cyanosis
Examine the conjunctivae, palms, soles, buccal mucosa, and tongue. Look for dull, dark color.

Edema
Examine the area for decreased color, and palpate for tightness.

Erythema
Palpate the area for warmth.

Jaundice
Examine the sclerae and hard palate in natural, not fluorescent, light if possible. Look for a yellow color.

Pallor
Examine the sclerae, conjunctivae, buccal mucosa, tongue, lips, nail beds, palms, and soles. Look for an ashen color.

Petechiae
Examine areas of lighter pigmentation such as the abdomen. Look for tiny, purplish red dots.

Rashes
Palpate the areas for skin texture changes.

■ Choose the best course

Insert the following steps in the proper sequence to show how you would conduct a skin, hair, and nail assessment.

Steps

Inspect and palpate hair, focusing on distribution, quantity, texture, and color.

Measure and note distribution of lesions.

Observe nail color, and press nail beds to assess peripheral circulation.

Inspect and palpate skin, focusing on color, texture, turgor, moisture, and temperature.

Assemble equipment, and put on gloves.

Observe skin's overall appearance.

Inspect nail shape and contour, and palpate nail bed for thickness and strength.

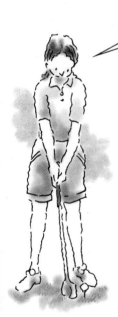

The best course on my day off is big and green and filled with lots of birdies.

Pep talk

" There is no need to go to India or anywhere else to find peace. You will find that deep place of silence right in your room, your garden, or even your bathtub. "
—Elisabeth Kübler-Ross

■ Match point

Match each type of primary lesion with its picture. As a bonus, also list one example of each lesion that you might find during a routine skin assessment.

1. _____
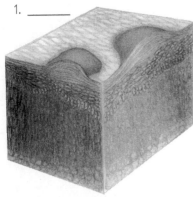

Bonus example: _____

2. _____
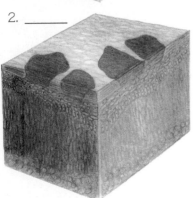

Bonus example: _____

3. _____
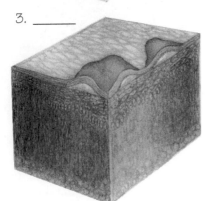

Bonus example: _____

Primary lesion

A. Macule

B. Papule

C. Vesicle

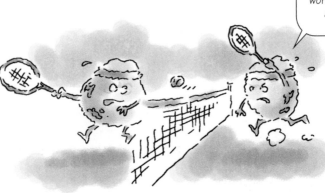

I'm sensing this is developing into more than a friendly workout—it's more like a grudge match!

Team colors

Complete the chart to have a full legion of lesion configurations for ready reference. Read each description carefully, and use a red pencil or marker to draw the missing patterns.

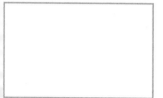

1. Discrete: Individual lesions are separate and distinct.

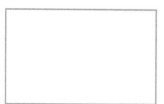

2. Grouped: Lesions are clustered together.

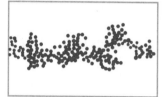

3. Confluent: Lesions merge so that individual lesions aren't visible or palpable.

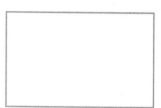

4. Linear: Lesions form a line.

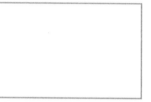

5. Annular: Lesions are arranged in a single ring or circle.

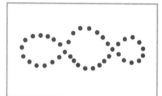

6. Polycyclic: Lesions are arranged in multiple circles.

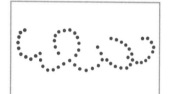

7. Arciform: Lesions form arcs or curves.

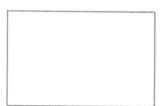

8. Reticular: Lesions form a meshlike network.

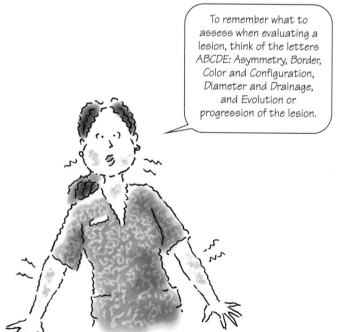

To remember what to assess when evaluating a lesion, think of the letters ABCDE: Asymmetry, Border, Color and Configuration, Diameter and Drainage, and Evolution or progression of the lesion.

■ Cross-training

Identify all of the common skin disorders in this puzzle and you'll be a force to contend with in the assessment arena.

Across

1. Hypopigmentation with irregular blotchiness on face, hands, and feet
4. Formed by permanently dilated, small blood vessels
9. Chronic disease characterized by plaques with silvery scales on scalp, elbows, and knees
10. Severe itching caused by mite infestation

Down

2. Facial rash that may result in oozing ruptured vesicles that crust over
3. Tinea corporis
5. Fungal infection that thrives in moist areas, such as under breasts and in axillae
6. Hives resulting from allergic reaction
7. Causes severe itching and dry skin, mostly affecting antecubital and popliteal areas
8. Butterfly-shaped rash on cheeks and nose

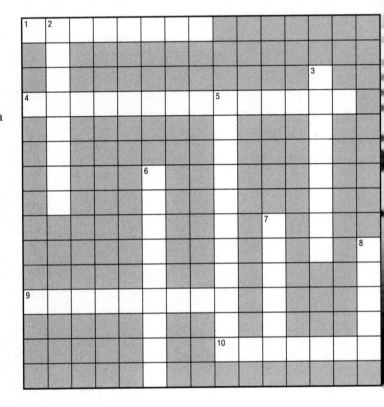

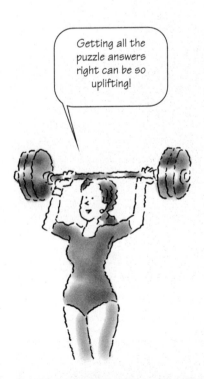

Getting all the puzzle answers right can be so uplifting!

Finish line

Sharpen your powers of observation by identifying the major fingernail structures shown in this illustration.

1._____

2._____

3._____

4._____

5._____

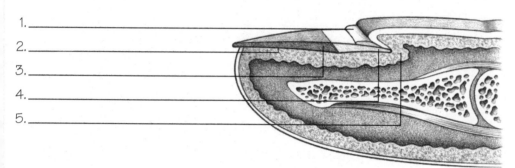

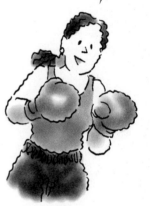

Here's one way to get in some necessary exercise—and protect your manicure at the same time!

You make the call

Identify which assessment finding is being evaluated in this illustration. Then explain the purpose of the test and the significance of the findings.

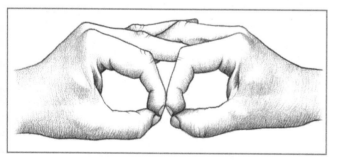

Assessment finding

_____

Significance

_____

_____

_____

_____

_____

■ Three-point conversion

Even Nurse Joy has her good days and her bad days... Identify which sign or symptom is best represented in each of the following illustrations.

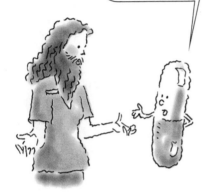

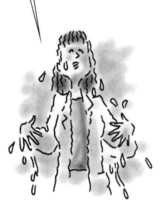

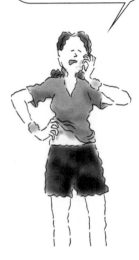

1. _____ 2. _____ 3. _____

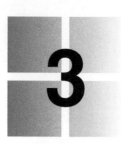

3

Neurologic system

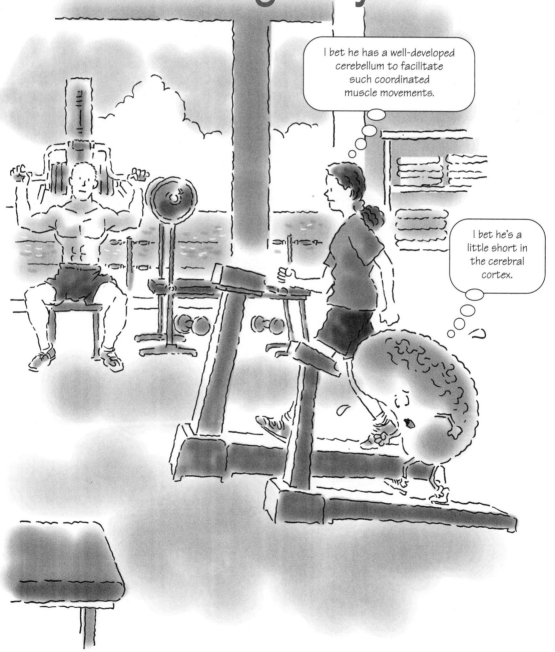

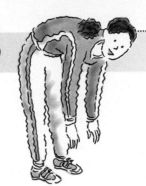

Neurologic system review

Central nervous system

Brain

■ Cerebrum (cerebral cortex): enables thinking and reasoning
■ Brainstem: acts as a major sensory and motor pathway for impulses to and from the cerebral cortex; regulates automatic body functions, such as heart rate and breathing
■ Cerebellum: facilitates coordinated muscle movement and maintains equilibrium

Spinal cord

■ Acts as the primary pathway for messages traveling between the peripheral areas of the body and the brain
■ Mediates the reflex arc

Peripheral nervous system

■ Peripheral nerves: serve the skin, muscles, sensory organs, and viscera
■ Cranial nerves: serve the brain, head, and neck

Autonomic nervous system

■ Regulates activities of the visceral organs
■ Affects smooth and cardiac muscles and glands
■ Consists of the sympathetic division (controls fight-or-flight reactions) and parasympathetic division (maintains baseline body functions)

The health history

■ Determine the patient's chief complaint, which may include headache, dizziness, faintness, confusion, impaired mental status, or balance or gait disturbances.
■ Ask about current health, including memory and ability to concentrate as well as current medications.
■ Ask about past health, including illnesses, accidents or injuries, surgeries, and allergies.
■ Inquire about a family history of neurologic disorders that may have a genetic component, such as seizures and migraine headaches.

Through complex and coordinated interactions, the three parts of the neurologic system — central, peripheral, and autonomic — integrate all physical, intellectual, and emotional activities. Pretty heady stuff, huh!

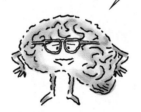

Assessment of mental status and speech

- Observe for any changes in level of consciousness.
- Note patient's appearance and behavior.
- Listen to how well patient speaks and expresses himself.
- Assess cognitive function by testing memory, orientation, attention span, calculation ability, thought content, abstract thinking, judgment, insight, and emotional status.
- Observe patient's constructional ability (ability to perform simple tasks and use various objects).

Assessment of cranial nerves

- Cranial nerve I (olfactory nerve): Have patient identify at least two scents.
- Cranial nerve II (optic nerve): Test visual acuity and visual fields with confrontation; examine fundus of the optic nerve.
- Cranial nerves III (oculomotor nerve), IV (trochlear nerve), and VI (abducent nerve): Test extraocular movement using the six cardinal positions of gaze.
- Cranial nerve V (trigeminal nerve): Check patient's ability to feel light touch and pain perception over face; have him clench his teeth to assess temporal and masseter muscles.
- Cranial nerve VII (facial nerve): Test taste perception; observe patient's face for symmetry at rest and when smiling, frowning, and raising eyebrows.

- Cranial nerve VIII (acoustic nerve): Test hearing and check balance.
- Cranial nerves IX (glossopharyngeal nerve) and X (vagus nerve): Check gag reflex.
- Cranial nerve XI (spinal accessory nerve): Check strength of sternocleidomastoid and trapezius muscles.
- Cranial nerve XII (hypoglossal nerve): Assess tongue position, movement, and strength; observe for tongue symmetry.

Assessment of sensory function

- Test pain perception in all dermatomes with sharp and dull ends of a safety pin.
- Test light touch sensation in all dermatomes using cotton wisp.
- Test vibratory sense with tuning fork over bony prominences.
- Assess position sense by having patient identify whether his toe or finger is positioned up or down as you move it.
- Assess discrimination by testing stereognosis, graphesthesia, and point localization.

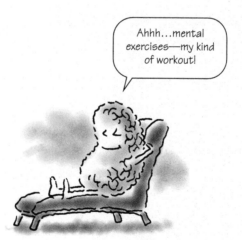

Ahhh...mental exercises—my kind of workout!

Assessment of motor function

- Assess muscle tone by guiding shoulders and hips through passive range-of-motion exercises.
- Assess muscle strength by having patient move major muscles and muscle groups against resistance.
- Assess cerebellar function by observing patient's coordination and general balance, testing extremity coordination, and having patient perform rapid alternating movements.

Assessment of reflexes

- Test deep tendon reflexes: biceps reflex, triceps reflex, brachioradialis reflex, patellar reflex, and Achilles reflex.
- Test superficial reflexes: Babinski's reflex (normally absent), cremasteric reflex (in males), and abdominal reflexes.
- Check for primitive reflexes (shouldn't be present in an adult but are normal in infants): grasp reflex, snout reflex, suck reflex, and glabella response.

Abnormal cranial nerve findings

- Olfactory impairment: inability to detect odors
- Visual impairment: visual field defects, pupillary changes, eye muscle impairment, and facial nerve impairment
- Auditory problems: difficulty hearing high-pitched sounds or total hearing loss
- Vertigo: illusion of movement resulting from a disturbance of vestibular centers
- Dysphagia: difficulty swallowing, typically after a stroke
- Speech disorders: impaired fluency or expression
- Constructional problems: apraxia (inability to perform purposeful movement) and agnosia (inability to identify common objects)

Abnormal muscle movements

- Tics: sudden uncontrolled movements of face, shoulders, and extremities
- Tremors: involuntary, repetitive movements in fingers, wrists, eyelids, tongue, and legs
- Fasciculations: fine twitchings in small muscle groups
- Abnormal gaits: spastic, scissors, propulsive, steppage, waddling

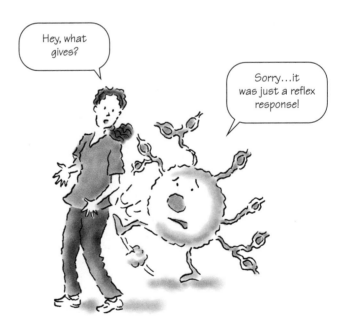

■ Batter's box

Test your knowledge of the neurologic system by filling in the blanks with the correct answers. Use each option only once.

Now, taking center stage

The central nervous system (CNS) includes the _____ and the
1

_____ . The _____ is the largest part of the brain; it
2   3

gives us the ability to think and reason and is divided into four _____
4

and two _____ .
5

The brainstem lies below the diencephalon, a division of the cerebrum, and is

divided into three parts: the _____ , _____ , and
6   7

_____ . The brainstem attaches to the spinal cord, which is the
8

primary pathway for messages traveling between the brain and peripheral areas; it

also mediates the sensory-to-motor transmission path known as the

_____ .
9

On the outskirts

The peripheral nervous system includes the peripheral and cranial

_____ . The _____ pairs of cranial nerves are the
10   11

primary _____ and _____ pathways between the brain
12   13

and the head and neck.

It's automatic

The autonomic nervous system consists of two parts: the sympathetic division,

which controls _____ reactions, and the parasympathetic division,
14

which maintains baseline body functions, such as _____ , heart rate,
15

swallowing, and coughing.

Options
brain

breathing

cerebrum

fight-or-flight

hemispheres

lobes

medulla

midbrain

motor

nerves

pons

reflex arc

sensory

spinal cord

12

I always try to
stay in shape—
sometimes that
adrenaline kicks in
when I least expect
it and off I go,
running for my life!

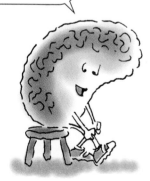

■ Match point

Match the cerebral lobe in column 1 with its function in column 2.

Cerebral lobe

1. Frontal lobe _____
2. Parietal lobe _____
3. Temporal lobe _____
4. Occipital lobe _____

Function

A. Sensations, awareness of body shape

B. Hearing, language and comprehension, storage and recall of memories

C. Personality, judgment, abstract reasoning, social behavior, language expression, movement

D. Visual stimuli

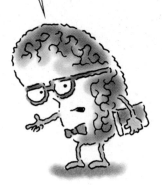

Don't look so nervous. It's only a simple matching game...not a mini-mental status exam!

■ Strikeout

Cross out the term that doesn't belong. Then, using the remaining words, identify the nervous system structure or component that's being assessed.

1. White matter, blue matter, gray matter, posterior horn, and anterior horn are all a part of the _____ _____ .

2. Level of consciousness, appearance and behavior, height and weight, speech, cognitive function, and constructional ability should be evaluated as part of a patient's _____ _____ .

3. Facial nerve, oculomotor nerve, olfactory nerve, radial nerve, and hypoglossal nerve are examples of _____ nerves.

4. Babinski's, brachioradialis, triceps, and Achilles are _____ _____ reflexes.

■ Finish line

Label the parts of the CNS illustrated in this cross section of the brain and spinal cord.

Brain

1. _____

2. _____

3. _____

4. _____

5. _____

6. _____

7. _____

8. _____

9. _____

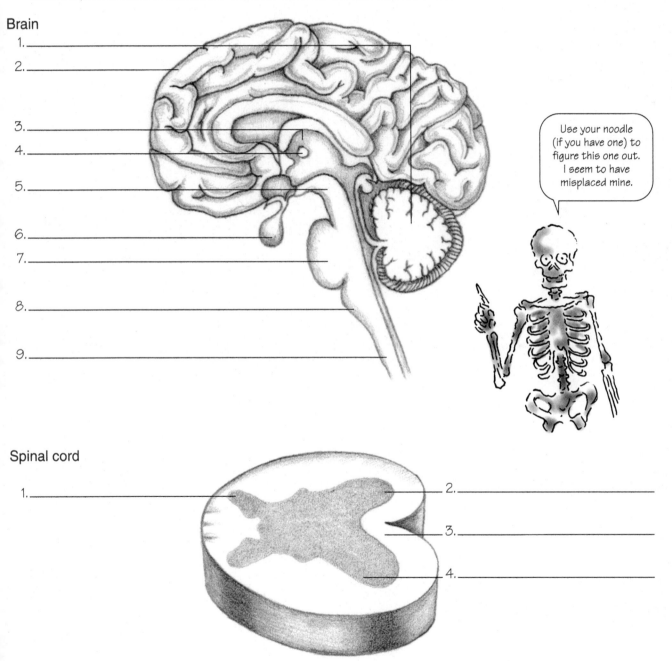

Use your noodle (if you have one) to figure this one out. I seem to have misplaced mine.

Spinal cord

1. _____

2. _____

3. _____

4. _____

Team colors

Trace the outline of the four lobes found in the cerebrum. Then color each lobe as follows: red (parietal lobe), blue (occipital lobe), yellow (temporal lobe), and green (frontal lobe).

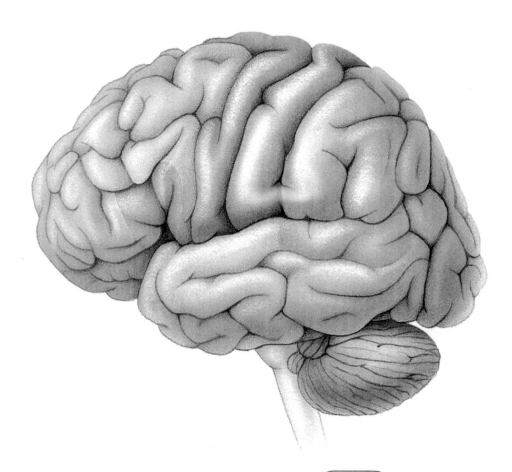

Pep talk

" Mind is the great leveler of all things; human thought is the process by which human ends are ultimately answered. "
—Daniel Webster

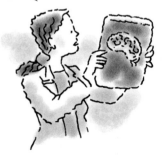

■ Train your brain

Sound out each group of pictures and symbols to reveal terms that complete this assessment consideration.

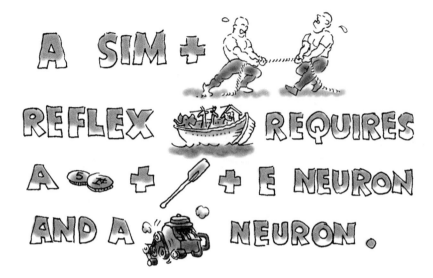

Answer: _____

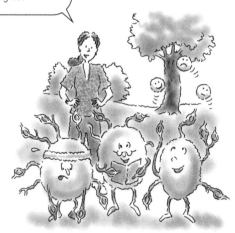

You make the call

Identify the physiologic process depicted in the illustration below. Then briefly describe how it occurs.

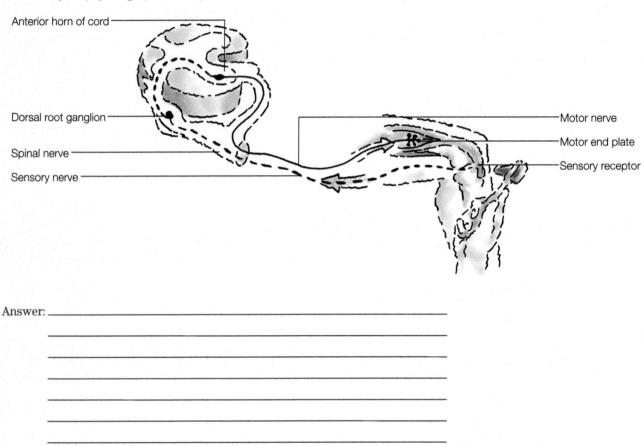

Anterior horn of cord

Dorsal root ganglion

Spinal nerve

Sensory nerve

Motor nerve

Motor end plate

Sensory receptor

Answer: _____

_____

_____

_____

_____

_____

_____

_____

_____

_____

_____

Brain crunches

List the seven most common complaints about the neurologic system reported by patients during a health history interview.

1. _____

2. _____

3. _____

4. _____

5. _____

6. _____

7. _____

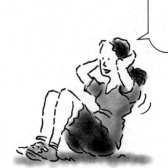

The one good thing about crunches...five...is that they're over...six...fairly quickly...seven. Whew!

Choose the best course

A neurologic examination is always conducted in an orderly fashion, beginning with the highest level of functioning and working down to the lowest. Fill in the boxes with these terms to show the proper sequence:

Steps

Motor function

Reflexes

Mental status and speech

Sensory function

Cranial nerve function

Match point

A quick mental status exam is an easy way to screen your patient for disordered thought processes. Match the question in column 1 with the function screened in column 2.

Question

1. Who's currently the U.S. president? _____
2. What's your name? _____
3. What year is it? _____
4. Where are you now? _____
5. What did you have for breakfast? _____
6. Can you count backward from 20 to 1? _____
7. What's your mother's name? _____
8. How old are you? _____
9. Where were you born? _____

Function screened

A. Remote memory

B. Orientation to other people

C. Memory

D. General knowledge

E. Attention span and calculation skills

F. Orientation to person

G. Orientation to place

H. Recent memory

I. Orientation to time

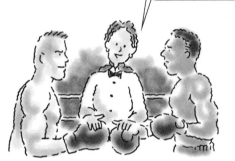

Being able to answer the question 'What's your name?' is a good way to decide on a TKO, too!

Train your brain

Sound out each group of pictures and symbols to reveal terms that complete this assessment consideration.

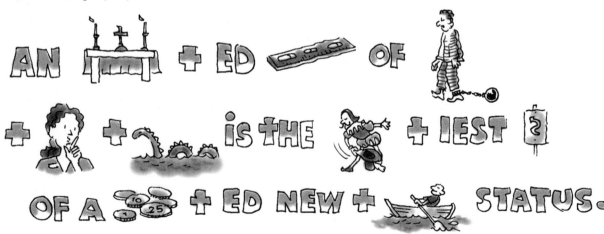

Answer: _____

■ Team up!

Write each assessment finding under the appropriate heading related to the mental status and speech portion of a neurologic examination.

Level of consciousness

_____

_____

_____

_____

_____

Appearance and behavior

_____

_____

_____

_____

_____

Speech

_____

_____

_____

_____

Cognitive function

_____

_____

_____

_____

Constructional ability

_____

_____

_____

_____

> You might want to conduct a more thorough mental status exam if your patient dresses like this and claims her mother's name is Anne Boleyn.

Findings
- Responds appropriately to hypothetical situation
- Confusion
- Poor grooming
- Poor attention span
- Dysarthria
- Lethargy
- Memory loss
- Inability to button clothing when asked
- Stuporousness
- Use of clanging
- Depression
- Opens eyes when told to
- Holds pencil but can't draw square
- Inappropriate clothes for season

■ Photo finish

Identify the postures shown in the illustrations below, and explain their significance in relation to the Glasgow Coma Scale.

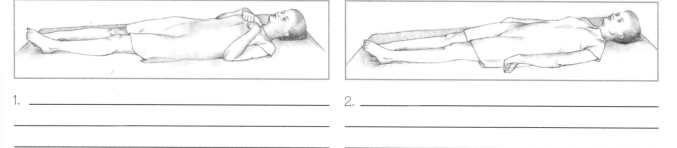

1. _____

_____

_____

2. _____

_____

_____

■ Hit or miss

Step up to the plate, and take a swing at whether the following statements about cranial nerve function are true or false.

_____ 1. Cranial nerve VII (cranial facial nerve) can be tested by placing various items on the tongue to test the patient's taste.

_____ 2. Cranial nerves III, IV, and V are usually all tested at the same time because they're related to ocular movement.

_____ 3. The acoustic nerve (cranial nerve VII) is responsible for hearing and equilibrium.

_____ 4. Tongue movement involved in swallowing and speech is controlled by the hypoglossal nerve (cranial nerve XII).

_____ 5. Cranial nerve I (olfactory nerve) is tested by having the patient identify such common substances as coffee and cinnamon.

_____ 6. Cranial nerve V is called the trigeminal nerve.

_____ 7. The glossopharyngeal nerve (cranial nerve IX) and vagus nerve (cranial nerve X) are tested together because their innervation overlaps in the nasal sinuses.

_____ 8. The optic nerve (cranial nerve II) is tested by having the patient read a newspaper and by a technique called confrontation.

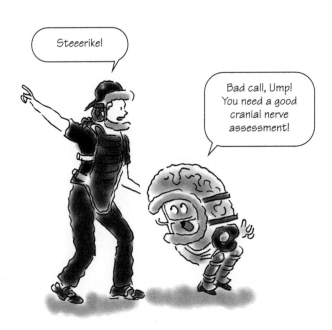

■ Match point

Match each sensation area listed with the image that shows the best assessment technique for evaluating it.

1. _____

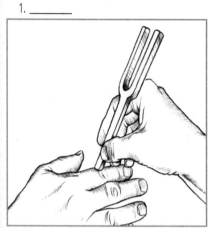

2. _____

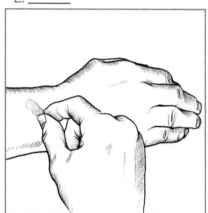

Assessment technique

A. Position

B. Light touch

C. Pain

D. Discrimination

E. Vibration

3. _____

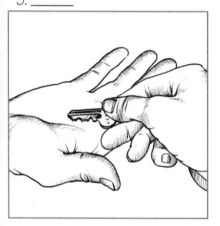

4. _____

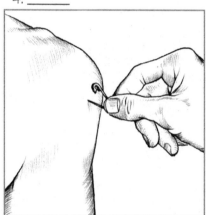

I'm not sure exactly what part of the sensory or motor system this evaluates, but it sure feels fun!

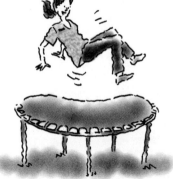

5. _____

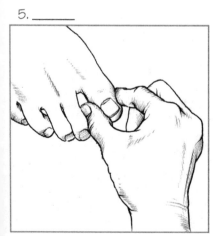

Jumble gym

Unscramble each term related to motor function evaluation. Then use the circled letters to answer the question.

Question: Besides muscles, what else should be tested when assessing a patient's motor system?
(*Hint:* It plays a role in smooth-muscle movements, such as tics, tremors, and fasciculations.)

1. DROSHULE LEGDRI _ _ _ _ _ _ _ _ _ _ _ _ _ ⃝ _

2. AGERN FO MOONIT _ _ _ ⃝ _ _ _ _ _ _ _ _ _ _

3. LUMCES NOTE _ _ _ _ ⃝ _ _ _ _ ⃝ _

4. GERMBORS SETT _ _ ⃝⃝ _ _ _ ' _ _ _ _ _ _

5. TINDOORCIAON ⃝ _ _ _ _ _ _ _ _ _ _ _

6. CLUEMS NESTGRHT _ ⃝ _ _ _ ⃝ _ _ ⃝ _ _ _ _ _

Answer: _ _ _ _ _ _ _ _ _

Let's see if this helps unscramble my brain a bit!

Brain crunches

Here's another quick mind-bender.

Question: Can you name five simple ways, besides Romberg's test, to assess your patient's coordination and general balance?

1. _____

2. _____

3. _____

4. _____

5. _____

You make the call

Identify the deep tendon reflex being tested in each illustration.

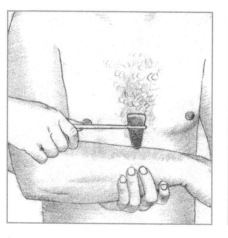

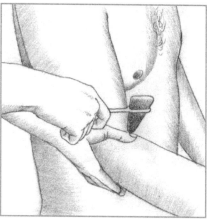

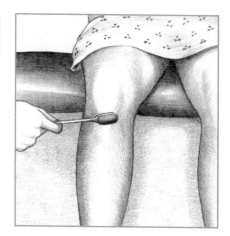

1. _____

2. _____

3. _____

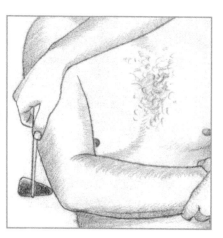

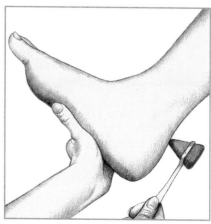

4. _____

5. _____

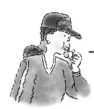

Coaching session

Testing deep tendon reflexes

The key to testing deep tendon reflexes is to make sure the patient is relaxed and the joint is flexed appropriately. First, distract the patient by asking him to focus on a point across the room. Always test deep tendon reflexes by moving from head to toe and comparing side to side.

Brain crunches

Just to keep you on your toes, here's another quick mind trick.

Question: **What are the four most common categories of abnormalities detected during a neurologic assessment?**

1. _____
2. _____
3. _____
4. _____

Match point

Match the deep tendon reflex scale number in column 1 with its corresponding response in column 2.

Reflex scale number

1. 0 _____
2. +1 _____
3. +2 _____
4. +3 _____
5. +4 _____

Response

A. Increased impulses (may be normal)

B. Absent impulses

C. Hyperactive impulses

D. Normal impulses

E. Diminished impulses

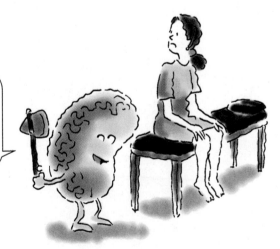

No, really...check it out! It's Ed McMahon with balloons and a giant check for 10 million dollars made out in your name...

◼◼ Cross-training

Here's an exercise to see how well your reflexes respond to horizontal and vertical clues.

Across

4. Elicited by applying gentle pressure to the palm

5. Normal reaction causes testicle to elevate

7. Elicited by striking tendon located on inside of elbow

9. Response elicited by repeatedly tapping bridge of nose

10. Common reflex in advanced dementia

11. Stroking from periphery toward midline stimulates umbilicus

12. Abnormal reflex that causes upward movement of big toe and fanning of little toes

Down

1. Deep tendon reflex elicited by striking above the olecranon process

2. Good flexion indicated by quadriceps contraction and leg extension

3. Striking the radium with a hammer causes this reflex

6. Striking this tendon causes plantar flexion of foot at the ankle

8. Pursing of lip after light tap on upper lip indicates frontal lobe damage

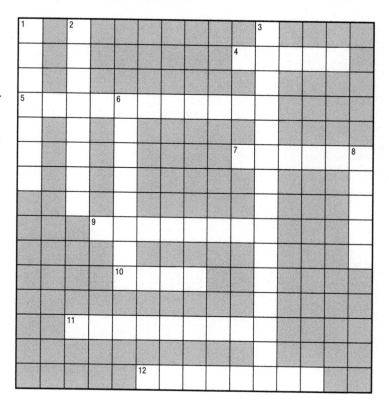

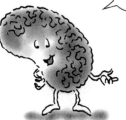

It suddenly crossed my mind that we haven't had a crossword puzzle yet in this chapter...enjoy!

Team up!

Write each assessment finding under the appropriate heading to indicate whether it's an early or late sign of increased intracranial pressure.

Early signs

_____

_____

_____

_____

_____

_____

_____

_____

_____

_____

_____

Late signs

_____

_____

_____

_____

_____

_____

_____

_____

_____

_____

_____

Findings
- Profound weakness
- Pupil changes on side of lesion
- Subtle orientation loss
- Sudden quietness
- Positive pronator drift (with palms up, one hand pronates)
- Sudden weakness
- Pupils fixed and dilated or "blown"
- Restlessness and anxiety
- Unarousable
- Motor changes on side opposite lesion
- One pupil constricts but then dilates (unilateral hippus)
- Requires increased stimulation
- Intermittent increases in blood pressure
- Sluggish reaction of both pupils
- Increased systolic pressure, profound bradycardia, abnormal respirations (Cushing's triad)

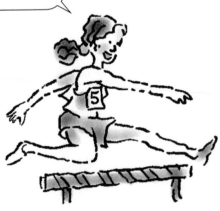

After this 4 x 100 relay, I'll never look at a 4 x 4 gauze pad the same way again!

Hit or miss

Indicate whether the following statements are true or false.

_____ 1. Common signs of head trauma include sudden aphasia, blurred or double vision, headache, cerebrospinal otorrhea or rhinorrhea, disorientation, behavior changes, and increased intracranial pressure.

_____ 2. Broca's aphasia is a form of receptive aphasia.

_____ 3. Agnosia is the inability to identify common objects.

_____ 4. A patient with ideation apraxia can perform simple activities but can't understand their effects.

_____ 5. Vertigo and dysphagia can indicate cranial nerve damage.

_____ 6. Like tics, tremors are involuntary, repetitive movements usually seen in the fingers, wrist, eyelids, tongue, and legs.

_____ 7. Damage to the peripheral labyrinth, brainstem, or cerebellum can cause nystagmus.

_____ 8. Global aphasia is the common name for Wernicke's aphasia.

_____ 9. Reflexes can be grouped into three major groups, including deep tendon reflexes, superficial reflexes, and primitive reflexes.

_____ 10. Fasciculations, fine twitchings involving small muscle groups, are most commonly associated with upper motor neuron dysfunction.

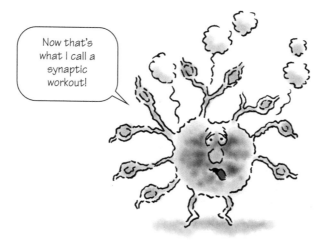

Winner's circle

Test your ability to assess and differentiate pupillary changes during a neurologic evaluation.

1. Circle the picture that shows unilateral dilated pupils.

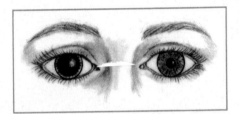 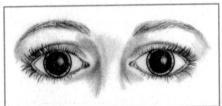

2. Circle the picture that shows bilateral pinpoint pupils.

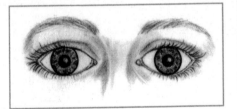 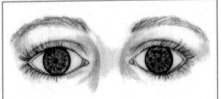

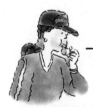

Coaching session
Look for pupil changes

If the patient's pupillary response to light is affected, he may have damage to the optic nerve and oculomotor nerve. Pupils are also a sensitive indicator of neurologic dysfunction. Increased intracranial pressure causes dilation of the pupil ipsilateral to the mass lesion; without treatment, both pupils become fixed and dilated. Having unequal pupils, or *anisocoria*, is normal in about 20% of people. In normal anisocoria, pupil size doesn't change.

4

Eyes

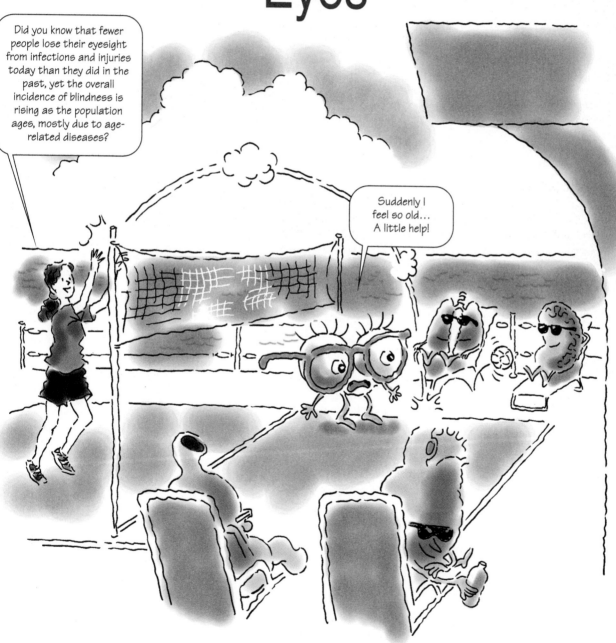

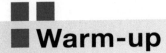
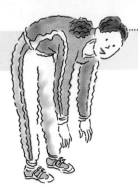

Eye review

Eye structures and functions

- Sclera—maintains the eye's size and shape
- Choroid—maintains blood supply to the eye
- Vitreous humor—maintains the placement of the retina and the eyeball's spherical shape
- Cornea—refracts, or bends, light rays entering the eye
- Iris—contains pigment granules that give the eye its color; contains involuntary muscles that control pupil size
- Pupil—permits light to enter the eye
- Lens—refracts and focuses light onto the retina
- Retina—receives visual stimuli and transmits images to the brain for processing

Health history

- Determine patient's chief complaint.
- Ask if patient wears corrective lenses.
- Obtain past medical history. Be sure to ask about disorders that may affect vision, such as hypertension, diabetes, or stroke.
- Ask about a family history of glaucoma, cataracts, or vision loss.
- Obtain a medication history. Some medications, such as digoxin (Lanoxin), can affect vision.
- Ask patient with vision impairment how he manages activities of daily living and assess his support system.

Assessment

- Note the position of the eyes.
- Check eyelids for closure and for redness, edema, inflammation, and lesions.
- Inspect for excessive tearing or dryness.
- Palpate the nasolacrimal sac.
- Examine the bulbar and palpebral conjunctiva.
- Inspect the cornea and assess corneal sensitivity using a wisp of cotton.
- Evaluate each iris for size, color, and shape.
- Examine the pupils for equal size, shape, and reactivity.

Tests for visual acuity

- Snellen chart, Snellen E chart, and near-vision chart—test near and distance vision and measure visual acuity
- Confrontation—tests peripheral vision and assesses visual fields

Tests for extraocular muscle function

- Corneal light reflex—light should fall at the same spot on each cornea
- Cardinal positions of gaze—eyes should remain parallel and move smoothly through the six cardinal positions
- Cover-uncover test—eye shouldn't move while covering or uncovering it

Ophthalmoscopic examination

- Have patient remove his corrective lenses; darken the room.
- Check for presence and depth of the red reflex.
- Examine the lens for clouding, foreign matter, or opacities.
- Examine the retina: Observe the vitreous body for clarity; note the characteristics of the blood vessels; identify the optic disk, noting color, shape, and borders; and locate the light-sensitive macula.

Abnormal findings

- Arteriolar narrowing—arterioles of the inner eye narrow to a width of about one-half that of vein width
- Decreased visual acuity—the inability to see clearly
- Diplopia—double vision
- Discharge—excretion of any substance other than tears
- Pain—may demand immediate attention
- Periorbital edema—swelling around the eyes
- Ptosis—a drooping upper eyelid
- Strabismus—eyes deviate from their normal gazing position
- Vision loss—may be central or peripheral
- Visual floaters—specks of varying shape and size that float through the visual field but disappear when the patient tries to look at them
- Visual halos—rings or halos seen when looking at bright lights

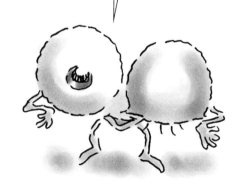

■ Batter's box

Stretch your memory and test your knowledge of eye anatomy and physiology by filling in the blanks with the appropriate words.

Losing sight of it all

Primary causes of vision loss include _____ , glaucoma,
₁

_____ , and macular degeneration—conditions that are
₂

more common among _____ patients. Younger patients
₃

can lose their sight from infections associated with HIV and AIDS as

well as from such opportunistic infections as _____ and
₄

_____ retinitis. Other vision disorders that can
₅

limit a person's ability to function include _____ ,
₆

_____ , and refractory errors.
₇

Ins and outs of eye structure

Extraocular structures include the bony orbits, which protect the eyes

from trauma, and the _____ , _____ ,
₈   ₉

and lacrimal apparatus, which protect the eyes from injury, dust, and

foreign bodies. Some of the essential intraocular structures include

the _____ , which refracts light rays entering the eye,
₁₀

the _____ , which is located in the center of the pupil,
₁₁

and the _____ , which receives visual stimuli and
₁₂

transmits images to the brain. Additionally, the eyes contain six

extraocular _____ innervated by the
₁₃

_____ , which control the movement of the eyes.
₁₄

Options

amblyopia

cataracts

cornea

cranial nerves

cytomegalovirus

diabetic retinopathy

elderly

eyelids

iris

lashes

retina

muscles

strabismus

toxoplasmosis

Two major benefits of a good mind stretch: to clear out the cobwebs from your brain and keep you on your toes.

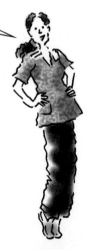

■ Match point

Who knew so many structures could fit inside one little eyeball? Match the intraocular structure in column 1 with its description in column 2.

Intraocular structure

1. Pupil _____
2. Lens _____
3. Vitreous chamber _____
4. Iris _____
5. Retina _____
6. Sclera _____
7. Cornea _____
8. Bulbar conjunctiva _____
9. Optic disk _____
10. Choroid _____
11. Ciliary body _____
12. Anterior chamber _____
13. Photoreceptor neurons _____

Description

A. Thin, transparent membrane that lines the eyelid

B. Innermost region of the eyeball that receives visual stimuli

C. Area just beneath iris that continuously produces aqueous humor

D. Smooth, avascular, transparent tissue located in front of the pupil and iris that refracts light rays and is associated with the protective blink reflex

E. Area filled with varying amounts of clear aqueous humor, which maintains pressure in the eye

F. Area lining the recessed portion of the eyeball that contains a network of vessels, which maintain blood supply to the back of the eye

G. White coating on the outside of the eyeball that helps maintain the eye's size and shape

H. Rod- or cone-shaped structures responsible for vision

I. Circular, contractile diaphragm that contains smooth and radial muscles and is perforated in the center by the pupil

J. Flexible structure located directly behind the iris that refracts and focuses light onto the retina

K. Central opening of the iris that allows light into the eye

L. Largest section of the eyeball filled with a thick, gelatinous substance that maintains placement of the retina and the eyeball's shape

M. "Blind spot" of eye where ganglion nerve axons exit the retina to form the optic nerve

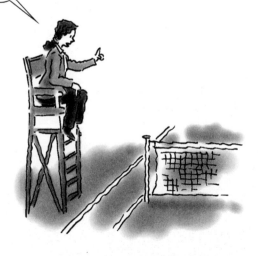

Quiet please... Miss Iris leads Miss Cornea two games to one.

■ Finish line

Focus now! Label each of the structures shown in this cross section of the eye.

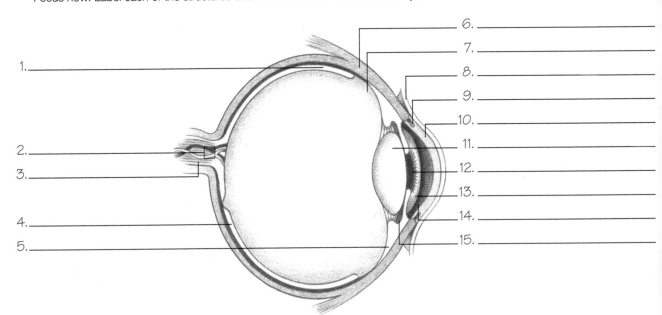

1. _____

2. _____
3. _____

4. _____
5. _____

6. _____
7. _____
8. _____
9. _____
10. _____
11. _____
12. _____
13. _____
14. _____
15. _____

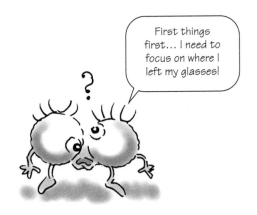

■ Brain crunches

Quick, now…What are the five most common eye-related complaints you're likely to hear when obtaining a health history?

1. _____
2. _____
3. _____
4. _____
5. _____

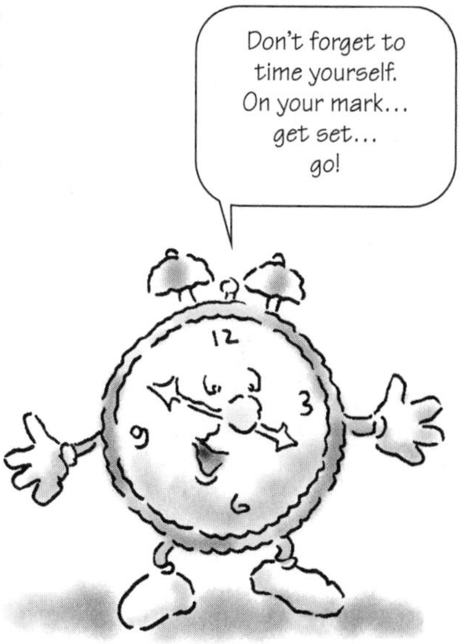

Don't forget to
time yourself.
On your mark…
get set…
go!

■ Mind sprints

Let's find out how far you can go in 5 minutes! Set your watch and see how
many questions you can ask your patient to obtain an accurate eye history.

_____
_____
_____
_____
_____
_____
_____
_____
_____
_____
_____
_____

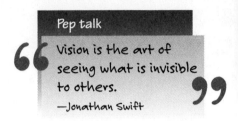

Pep talk

Vision is the art of seeing what is invisible to others.

—Jonathan Swift

Gear up!

Check off which equipment you should have on hand when preparing to conduct an eye examination.

☐ Stethoscope
☐ Lamp or other light source
☐ Ophthalmoscope
☐ Speculum
☐ Scale
☐ Measuring tape
☐ Safety pin
☐ Vision test cards
☐ Gloves
☐ Cotton-tipped applicators
☐ Tongue blade
☐ Tissues
☐ Penlight
☐ Opaque cards
☐ Otoscope
☐ Povidone-iodine solution
☐ Syringe and needle

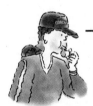

Coaching session
Modifying the health history interview

If your patient is a child or an older adult, you'll need to modify your health history to focus on some age-specific eye issues. Ask the parents (in the case of a child) or a family member or caregiver (if the older adult has difficulty remembering) to provide the information you need.

Child
• Was the child delivered vaginally or by cesarean birth? If vaginally, did his mother have a vaginal infection at the time? (Infections such as chlamydia, gonorrhea, genital herpes, or candidiasis can cause eye problems in infants.)
• Was erythromycin ointment instilled in his eyes at birth?
• Has he passed the normal developmental milestones?
• Does he know how to hold and care for sharp objects such as scissors?

Aging adult
• Have you had any difficulty climbing stairs or driving?
• Have you ever been tested for glaucoma? If so, when and what was the result?
• If you have glaucoma, has your doctor prescribed eyedrops for you? If so, what kind?
• How well can you instill your eyedrops?
• Do your eyes ever feel dry? Do they burn? If so, how do you treat the problem?

Match point

Match the eye structure in column 1 with the corresponding eye inspection technique in column 2.

Eye structure

1. Cornea _____

2. Eyelids _____

3. Pupils _____

4. Conjunctiva _____

5. Iris _____

Inspection technique

A. Hold eyelids either up or down, and inspect for color changes, foreign bodies, exudate, and edema

B. Observe for styes, excessive tearing or dryness, and entropion or ectropion

C. Check for flatness and symmetrical size, color, and shape

D. Check for symmetry, light reactivity, and accommodation

E. Use penlight to check for clarity, then a wisp of cotton for sensitivity

> It may seem cliché, but it's a winning technique: Always keep your eye on the ball!

You make the call

Identify the eye charts below, and describe why and for whom they're used.

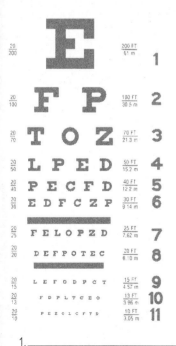

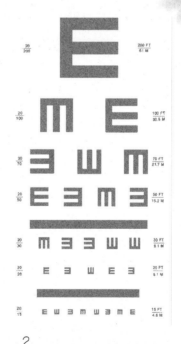

1. _____

_____

_____

_____

_____

2. _____

_____

_____

_____

_____

Three-point conversion

Identify what the nurse is assessing in each of the following illustrations.

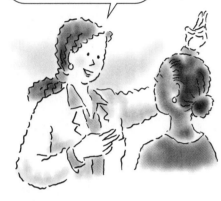

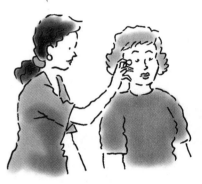

1. _____ 2. _____ 3. _____

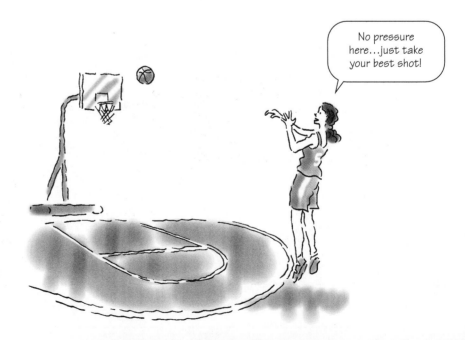

■ Hit or miss

Indicate whether the following statements are true or false.

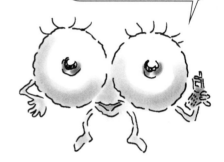

Eyeball these true-or-false statements and remember, if need be, you can always phone a friend as your last lifeline to get the correct answer.

_____ 1. Assessing the corneal light reflex and cardinal positions of gaze and performing the cover-uncover test are good ways to evaluate your patient's intraocular muscles.

_____ 2. A patient who lacks extraocular muscle coordination has a condition called strabismus.

_____ 3. An ophthalmoscope allows for direct observation of the eye's internal structures.

_____ 4. The blue reflex is a reflection of light off the choroid when viewed through an ophthalmoscope.

_____ 5. To test far vision, hold a Rosenbaum card 14″ (35.6 cm) from the patient's eyes and ask him to read the line with the smallest letters he can distinguish.

_____ 6. The macula is the part of the eye that's most sensitive to light.

_____ 7. A patient with an opaque lens most likely has cataracts.

_____ 8. When viewing retinal structures through an ophthalmoscope, veins appear thinner and brighter than arteries.

■ Winner's circle

Circle the picture that shows the correct way to position an ophthalmoscope to examine the eye's internal structures.

1.

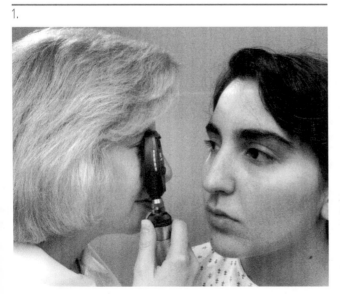

2.

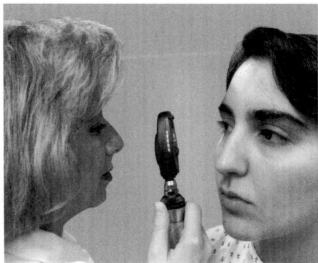

Team colors

First identify the retinal structures that appear in this illustration. Then, color the arterioles red and the veins blue.

Warning...Don't forget the second half of this two-part game!

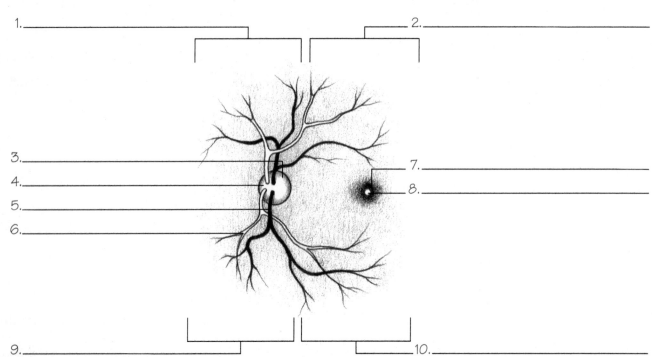

1. _____

2. _____

3. _____

4. _____

5. _____

6. _____

7. _____

8. _____

9. _____

10. _____

Pep talk

" For a clever eye, one glance is enough, while a dunce may stare all day long. "
—Chinese proverb

■ Mind sprints

Write the findings you'd expect to note when assessing a patient with the following conditions.
Time yourself, and see how many you can list in 5 minutes.

Bacterial conjunctivitis:

_____

_____

_____

_____

_____

_____

_____

Retinal detachment:

_____

_____

_____

_____

_____

_____

_____

Cataracts:

_____

_____

_____

_____

_____

_____

_____

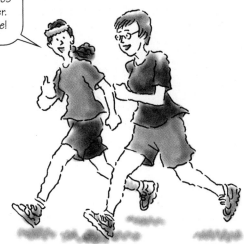

■ You make the call

Identify the abnormality shown in the pictures below.

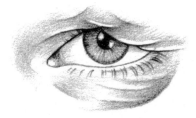

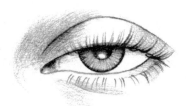

1. _____

2. _____

Match point

What's up with all those eye problems? Match the eye assessment finding in column 1 with the probable cause in column 2.

Assessment finding

1. Eye pain _____
2. Diplopia _____
3. Vision loss _____
4. Visual halos _____
5. Strabismus _____
6. Periorbital edema _____
7. Eye discharge _____
8. Ptosis _____
9. Visual floaters _____
10. Visual auras _____

Probable cause

A. Conjunctivitis, other inflammatory or infectious eye disorders, systemic disorders

B. Angle-closure glaucoma, conjunctivitis, foreign body, abrasions, trauma

C. Increased intraocular pressure, corneal edema, fluctuation in blood glucose levels

D. Small cells in vitreous humor, vitreous hemorrhage, retinal separation or detachment

E. Interruption in sympathetic innervation, muscle weakness, damage to the oculomotor nerve

F. Migraine headache

G. Allergies, local inflammation, fluid-retaining disorders, crying

H. Misaligned extraocular muscles

I. Extraocular weakness or paralysis, thyroid ophthalmology, retinoblastoma

J. Glaucoma, untreated cataracts, retinal disease, macular degeneration

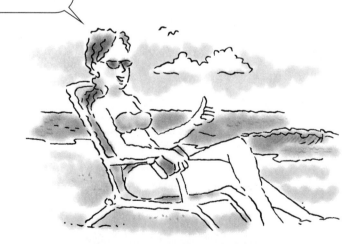

5

Ear, nose, and throat

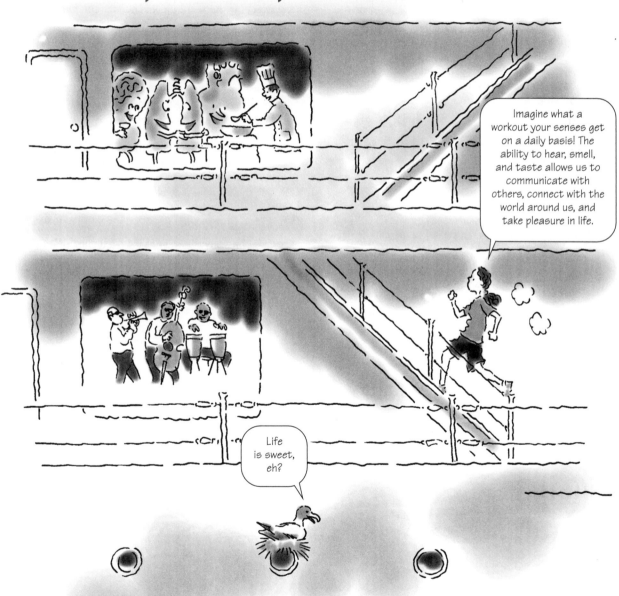
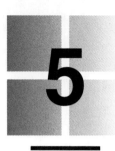

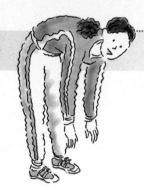

■ Warm-up

Ears, nose, and throat review

Health history

■ Ask about common ear complaints, such as hearing loss, tinnitus, pain, and dizziness.
■ Discuss past medical history, including allergies.
■ Ask about common nose complaints, such as nasal stuffiness, nasal discharge, and nosebleed.
■ Ask about colds, headaches, and sinus problems.
■ Ask about common throat complaints, such as bleeding or sore gums, sore throat, and tooth problems.
■ Ask the patient whether he smokes or uses other types of tobacco.
■ Ask about neck problems, such as neck pain, swelling, or trouble moving the neck.

Ear

EXTERNAL EAR

■ Consists mainly of elastic cartilage
■ Collects sounds and transmits them to the middle ear

MIDDLE EAR

■ Separated from the external ear by the tympanic membrane
■ Contains three small bones: the malleus, the incus, and the stapes
■ Connects to the nasopharynx via the eustachian tube
■ Transmits sound vibrations to the inner ear, protects the auditory apparatus, and equalizes air pressure on both sides of the tympanic membrane

INNER EAR

■ Consists of closed, fluid-filled spaces
■ Contains the vestibule and semicircular canals that help to maintain equilibrium, and the cochlea, the organ of hearing

Assessment

■ Observe the ears for position and symmetry.
■ Inspect the external ear for lesions, drainage, nodules, or redness.
■ Inspect and palpate the mastoid area behind each auricle.
■ Perform an otoscopic examination: examine the external canal, noting the presence and color of cerumen, and then advance the otoscope to view the tympanic membrane.
■ Use Weber's test to evaluate a patient with diminished or lost hearing in one ear.
■ Use the Rinne test to compare air conduction of sound with bone conduction of sound.

Abnormal findings

■ Earache—severity ranges from a feeling of fullness or blockage to deep, boring pain
■ Hearing loss—can be conductive or sensorineural
■ Otorrhea—drainage from the ear

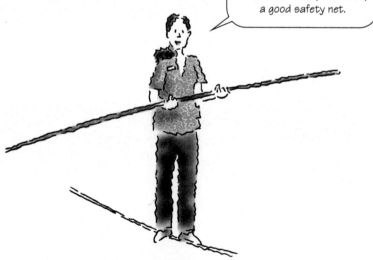

Kids, don't try this at home without a properly functioning inner and middle ear—and, of course, a good safety net.

Nose

- Acts as sensory organ of smell
- Filters, warms, and humidifies inhaled air
- Linked internally to four pairs of paranasal sinuses: maxillary (on the cheeks below the eyes), frontal (above the eyebrows), and ethmoidal and sphenoidal (behind the eyes and nose)

Assessment

- Observe the nose for position, symmetry, and color. Note nasal flaring or discharge.
- Test nasal patency and the olfactory nerve (cranial nerve I) by having the patient obstruct one nostril and identify a smell with the other.
- Inspect the nasal cavity using the light from the otoscope, checking the vestibule, turbinates, and nostrils.
- Palpate the nose for pain, tenderness, swelling, and deformity.
- Examine the frontal and maxillary sinuses (the only sinuses that are accessible for examination).
- Check for swelling around the eyes.
- Palpate the sinuses. Use transillumination, if necessary, to help reveal obstructions and tumors.

Abnormal findings

- Epistaxis—nosebleed; a common sign
- Nasal flaring—may be a sign of respiratory distress
- Nasal stuffiness and discharge—obstruction of the nasal mucous membranes along with a discharge of thin mucus

Throat and neck

- Consists of nasopharynx, oropharynx, and laryngopharynx
- Contains cervical vertebrae, the major neck and shoulder muscles, and their ligaments
- Contains trachea, thyroid gland, and chains of lymph nodes

Assessment

- Inspect the lips.
- Use a tongue blade and a bright light to inspect the oral mucosa, gingivae (gums), and teeth.
- Inspect the tongue and note the patient's ability to move it in all directions. Also inspect underneath the tongue.
- Inspect and palpate the neck.
- Assess lymph nodes.
- Palpate the trachea and thyroid gland.
- Auscultate the neck by listening over the carotid arteries and over the thyroid gland (if it's enlarged).

Abnormal findings

- Dysphagia—difficulty swallowing
- Throat pain—discomfort in any part of the pharynx; may range from a scratchy sensation to severe pain

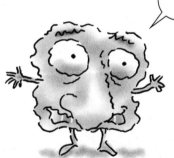

I'm picking up the scent of a challenging exercise or two around the next bend. Hope you're ready!

■■
■ Batter's box

Here's an anatomy and physiology pick-me-up to help get you started. Fill in the blanks with the appropriate words.

Hear ye, hear ye!

The external ear is made up of mainly elastic _____ and contains the ear
$\underline{\hspace{2cm}}_{1}$

flap, also known as the auricle or _____ , and the auditory canal. The
$\underline{\hspace{2cm}}_{2}$

_____ membrane separates the external and middle ear. The middle ear, a
$\underline{\hspace{2cm}}_{3}$

small, air-filled structure that transmits _____ vibrations to the inner ear,
$\underline{\hspace{2cm}}_{4}$

connects with the _____ , which keeps nasopharyngeal contaminants from
$\underline{\hspace{2cm}}_{5}$

entering the normally sterile ear environment. Besides controlling hearing, the structures

in the middle and inner ear work to control a person's _____ .
$\underline{\hspace{2cm}}_{6}$

The nose knows

More than just the sensory organ of _____ , the nose plays a key role in the
$\underline{\hspace{2cm}}_{7}$

_____ system by filtering, warming, and _____ inhaled air.
$\underline{\hspace{2cm}}_{8}$ $\underline{\hspace{2cm}}_{9}$

The internal and external portions of the nose are divided by the nasal

_____ . Four pairs of _____ open into the internal nose and
$\underline{\hspace{2cm}}_{10}$ $\underline{\hspace{2cm}}_{11}$

serve as resonators for sound production and provide _____ .
$\underline{\hspace{2cm}}_{12}$

Deep throat and beyond

The throat is divided into the _____ , _____ , and
$\underline{\hspace{2cm}}_{13}$ $\underline{\hspace{2cm}}_{14}$

_____ . It contains the hard and soft
$\underline{\hspace{2cm}}_{15}$

_____ , the uvula, and the _____ .
$\underline{\hspace{2cm}}_{16}$ $\underline{\hspace{2cm}}_{17}$

The _____ is formed by the cervical vertebrae, the
$\underline{\hspace{2cm}}_{18}$

major neck and shoulder muscles, and their ligaments. It contains

the butterfly-shaped _____ gland, which produces
$\underline{\hspace{2cm}}_{19}$

the hormones _____ and thyroxine.
$\underline{\hspace{2cm}}_{20}$

Options
balance
cartilage
eustachian tube
humidifying
laryngopharynx
mucus
nasopharynx
neck
oropharynx
palates
paranasal sinuses
pinna
respiratory
septum
smell
sound
thyroid
tonsils
triiodothyronine
tympanic

> The unmistakable smell of coffee in the morning...now that's what I call a pick-me-up!

Cross-training

Stretch your brain muscles across and down with this anatomical crossword puzzle.

Across

2. Hairlike structures in inner ear that respond to body movement

4. Gland located in anterior neck, just below the larynx

5. Throat

7. Area that's common site of nosebleeds

10. Nostrils

11. Type of tissue found in much of ear and nose

13. Sinuses assessed along with nose

14. How sound waves are conducted

16. Fluid filling the space between bony labyrinth and membranous labyrinth

17. Divides the nose vertically

Down

1. Membrane also known as the eardrum

2. One of three structures composing bony labyrinth

3. Maxillary, frontal, ethmoidal, or sphenoidal

6. One of three bones in middle ear

8. Tube connecting middle ear with pharynx

9. Region of nose rich in capillaries and mucus-producing goblet cells

12. Other word for pinna

15. Protrusion hanging from roof of mouth

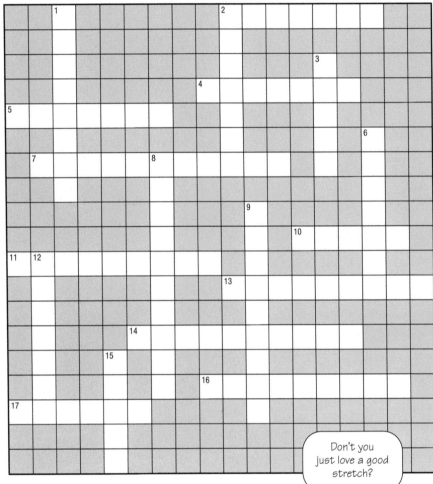

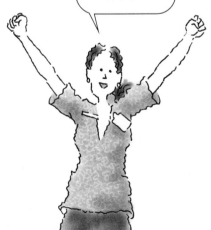

Don't you just love a good stretch?

■■
■ Finish line

Identify the external, middle, and inner ear structures illustrated below.

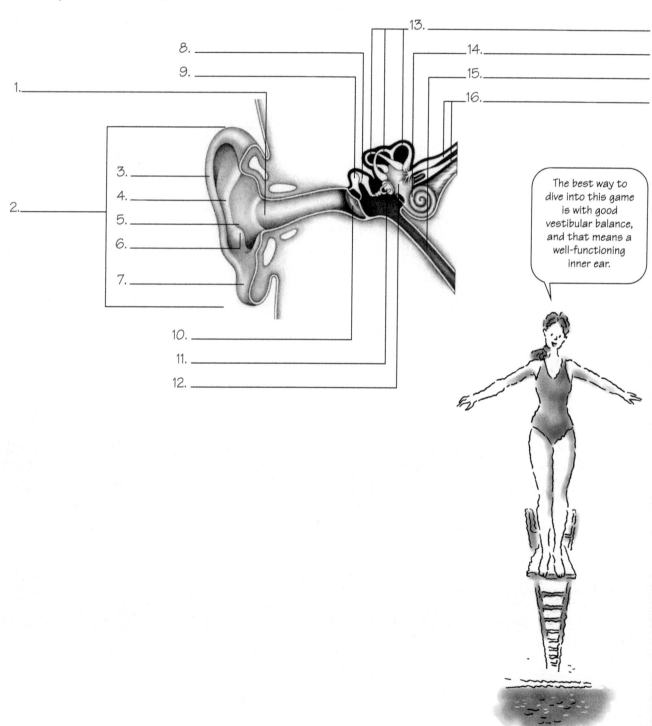

8. _____

9. _____

13. _____

14. _____

15. _____

16. _____

1. _____

2. _____

3. _____

4. _____

5. _____

6. _____

7. _____

10. _____

11. _____

12. _____

The best way to dive into this game is with good vestibular balance, and that means a well-functioning inner ear.

■ Brain crunches

Listen up, and think fast! List the five most common ear complaints reported during the health history.

1._____
2._____
3._____
4._____
5._____

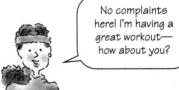

No complaints here! I'm having a great workout—how about you?

■ Mind sprints

See if you can go the distance by listing questions you should ask your patient about his chief complaint of "ear problems." Time yourself, and see how many questions you can list in 5 minutes.

_____
_____
_____
_____
_____
_____
_____
_____
_____
_____

Pep talk

" If a man does not keep pace with his companions, perhaps it is because he hears a different drummer. Let him keep step to the music he hears, however measured and far away. "
—Henry David Thoreau

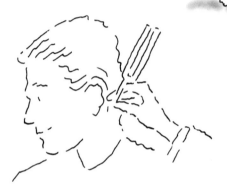

Ommmmmmmmm… In case you're wondering, my mantra's tuned to 512 cycles/second—the same as my tuning fork.

■■
■ You make the call

Identify the test shown in each illustration, and describe why it's being done.

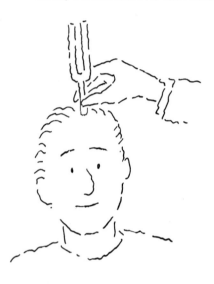

1. _____

_____

_____

_____

_____

2. _____

_____

_____

_____

_____

■■
■ Hit or miss

Listen up and you'll do fine with this game! Indicate whether the following statements about ear examinations are true or false.

_____ 1. Low-set ears are a common finding in patients with congenital disorders.

_____ 2. Cerumen is normally dry and flaky in Blacks and Whites, and dark brown and moist in Asians and Native Americans.

_____ 3. Displacement or absence of the light reflex may be due to a bulging, inflamed, or retracted tympanic membrane.

_____ 4. A patient who hears a tone in his unaffected ear while a Weber's test is being conducted means he has a conductive hearing loss.

_____ 5. Hearing in an infant or young child is commonly tested by assessing the startle reflex.

_____ 6. The correct way to straighten an adult's ear canal before inserting a speculum is to pull the auricle down and sideways.

_____ 7. When viewed through an otoscope, the tympanic membrane should appear pink, dry, and opaque.

■■
■ Team colors

Get out your colored pencils for this one. First, identify the tympanic membrane structures you'd see through an otoscope as illustrated below. Then, color the annulus yellow and the light reflex blue. (*Hint:* We've just given away two of the answers.)

1. _____

2. _____

3. _____

4. _____

5. _____

6. _____

7. _____

■■
■ Match point

Who said an ears, nose, and throat exam can't be fun? Match the assessment technique in column 1 with its corresponding procedure in column 2.

Assessment technique

1. Palpating maxillary sinuses _____

2. Testing nasal patency _____

3. Palpating frontal sinuses _____

4. Palpating thyroid _____

5. Palpating lymph nodes _____

Procedure

A. Place thumbs above eyes and fingertips on forehead, then apply gentle pressure

B. Place fingers around patient's neck from behind and ask him to swallow

C. Press thumbs on each side of nose just below cheekbones

D. Use finger pads to feel bilaterally under the patient's chin, then under and behind the ears

E. Block one nostril, and have patient inhale familiar aromatic substance through other nostril

This one's not on the matching test, but I'm sure you'll be able to figure out the technique...Place two hands on tired, achy muscles, rub gently, and listen for contented sigh!

■ Finish line

Identify the nose and mouth structures shown in the illustrations below.

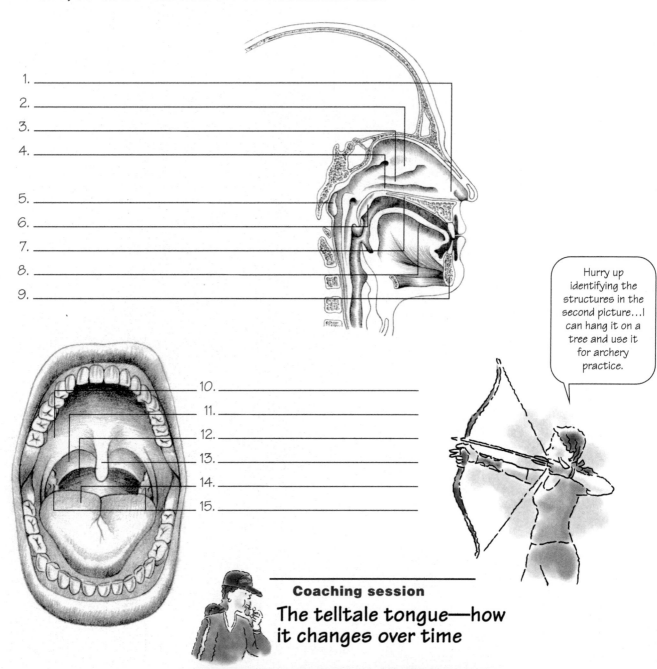

1. _____
2. _____
3. _____
4. _____

5. _____
6. _____
7. _____
8. _____
9. _____

10. _____
11. _____
12. _____
13. _____
14. _____
15. _____

Hurry up identifying the structures in the second picture...I can hang it on a tree and use it for archery practice.

Coaching session

The telltale tongue—how it changes over time

When assessing an older patient's oral cavity, look for varicose veins on the ventral surface of the tongue. Also, be aware that the area underneath the tongue is a common site for the development of oral cancers. This area must be assessed thoroughly.

You make the call

Identify which assessment technique is being performed in this illustration, and explain why it's being done.

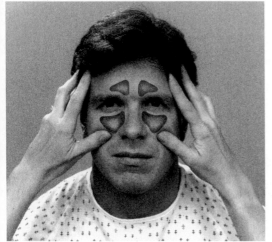

_____
_____
_____
_____
_____
_____
_____
_____
_____
_____

Team colors

First identify the lymph nodes pictured in the illustration, then color or circle all of the cervical nodes. This one is a little harder than it looks. (*Hint:* There are several cervical nodes, but they aren't all in a row.)

1. _____
2. _____
3. _____

7. _____
8. _____
9. _____
10. _____

4. _____
5. _____

6. _____

■■
■ Batter's box

Fill in the blanks with the correct words and you'll have a handy checklist of some of the most common abnormalities detected during an ears, nose, and throat assessment.

Options
cerumen (ear wax)

cold

ear

eardrum

epistaxis

esophageal

laryngitis

middle ear

nasal flaring

sinuses

■ _____ , another name for a nosebleed, can occur spontaneously or be
₁
induced from the front or back of the nose.

■ Otorrhea, or drainage from the _____ , may be bloody, purulent, clear,
₂
or sanguineous.

■ Dysphagia, or difficulty swallowing, is the most common symptom of

_____ disorders.
₃

■ Marked, regular _____ in an adult may signal respiratory distress.
₄

■ Mild to severe hoarseness, accompanied by temporary loss of voice, malaise,

low-grade fever, dysphagia, dry cough, and tender or enlarged cervical lymph nodes, is

probably caused by _____ .
₅

■ Serous otitis media, another name for inflammation of the _____ , is
₆
common in those with seasonal allergies.

■ Acute otitis media is characterized by severe, deep, throbbing pain, hearing loss, high

fever, and a bulging, fiery red _____ .
₇

■ Impacted _____ can cause a sensation of fullness in the ear, itching,
₈
partial hearing loss, and possible dizziness; it should never be removed with an

instrument because it can cause the patient excessive pain.

■ Thick, purulent drainage, fever, and severe pain over the _____ usually
₉
indicate sinusitis.

■ A patient with watery nasal discharge, sneezing, temporary loss of smell and taste,

sore throat, malaise, arthralgia, and mild headache most likely has a common

_____ .
₁₀

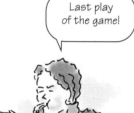

Last play
of the game!

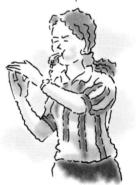

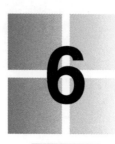

6

Cardiovascular system

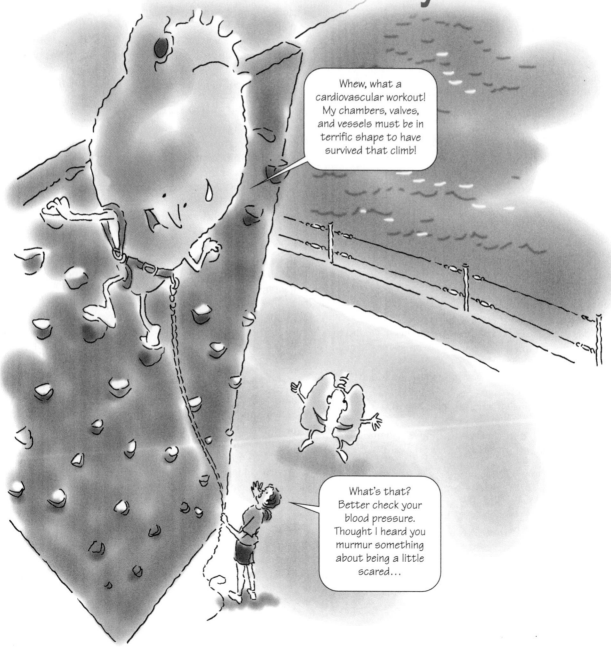

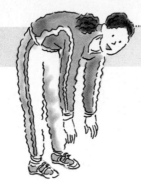
Cardiovascular system review

Structures

Heart

■ A hollow, muscular organ that pumps blood to all organs and tissues of the body
■ Protected by a thin sac called the *pericardium*
■ Consists of four chambers: two atria and two ventricles
■ Contains valves to keep blood flowing in only one direction
■ Contracts to send blood out (systole), then relaxes and fills with blood (diastole)

Vascular system

■ Arteries: thick-walled vessels that carry oxygenated blood away from the heart
■ Veins: thin-walled vessels that carry deoxygenated blood toward the heart
■ Pulses: pressure waves of blood generated by the pumping action of the heart

Blood circulation

■ Deoxygenated venous blood flows from the superior vena cava, inferior vena cava, and coronary sinus into the right atrium.
■ Blood flows from the right atrium through the tricuspid valve and into the right ventricle.
■ Blood is then ejected through the pulmonic valve into the pulmonary artery, where it travels to the lungs for oxygenation.
■ Oxygenated blood then flows through the pulmonary veins and returns to the left atrium.
■ Blood passes through the mitral valve and into the left ventricle.
■ Blood is pumped through the aortic valve and into the aorta for delivery to the rest of the body.

Obtaining a health history

■ Ask about current problems, including chest pain, palpitations, shortness of breath, peripheral skin changes, and changes in extremities.
■ Have the patient rate his chest pain on a scale of 0 to 10, with 0 being no pain and 10 being the worst pain imaginable.
■ Ask about a family history of cardiovascular disease, diabetes, and chronic diseases of the lungs or kidneys.

Assessing the heart

■ Inspect the patient's general appearance, noting skin color, temperature, turgor, and texture.
■ Inspect the chest, noting the location of the apical impulse.
■ Palpate over the precordium to find the apical impulse.
■ Palpate the sternoclavicular, aortic, pulmonic, tricuspid, and epigastric areas for abnormal pulsations.
■ Percuss the chest wall to locate cardiac borders.
■ Auscultate for heart sounds with the patient lying on his back with the head of the bed raised 30 to 45 degrees, with him sitting up, and with him lying on his left side.
■ Auscultate for murmurs by asking the patient to sit up and lean forward or having him lie on his left side.
■ Auscultate for a pericardial friction rub by asking the patient to sit upright, lean forward, and exhale.

Heart sounds

■ S_1: best heard at the apex of the heart; corresponds to closure of the mitral and tricuspid valves
■ S_2: best heard at the base of the heart; corresponds to closure of the pulmonic and aortic valves
■ S_3: commonly heard in patients with high cardiac output or heart failure (called *ventricular gallop*); a normal finding in children and young adults
■ S_4: adventitious sound called *atrial gallop;* heard in patients who are elderly or in those with hypertension, aortic stenosis, or a history of myocardial infarction

Assessing the vascular system

▪ Inspect the patient's general appearance, skin, and fingernails and toenails.
▪ Check the carotid artery pulsations and the jugular venous pulse.
▪ Palpate the patient's skin over the upper and lower extremities for temperature, texture, and turgor.
▪ Check capillary refill time (should be less than 3 seconds).
▪ Palpate arterial pulses on each side of the body, moving from head-to-toe (temporal, carotid, brachial, radial, femoral, popliteal, posterior tibial, and dorsalis pedis arteries, in that order).
▪ Auscultate over each artery in this same order, listening for hums or bruits.

Abnormal findings

▪ Chest pain: sensation that varies in severity and presentation depending on the cause
▪ Palpitations: a conscious awareness of one's heartbeat
▪ Fatigue: a feeling of excessive tiredness, lack of energy, or exhaustion accompanied by a strong desire to rest or sleep
▪ Thrill: palpable vibration indicating valvular dysfunction
▪ Heave: lifting of the chest wall felt during palpation; indicates ventricular hypertrophy (when felt on the sternal border) or ventricular aneurysm (when felt over the left ventricle)
▪ Murmur: sound made by turbulent blood flow; may increase in intensity (crescendo) or decrease in intensity (decrescendo)
▪ Bruit: a murmurlike sound heard over blood vessels

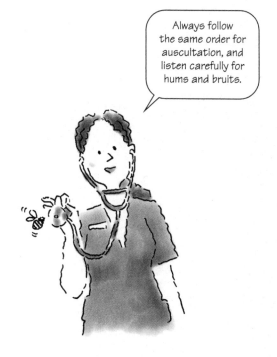

■ Batter's box

Test your familiarity with the anatomy and physiology of the cardiovascular system by filling in the blanks with the appropriate words.

What a system!

The cardiovascular system delivers _____ blood to tissues and removes

_____ . The _____ nervous system controls how the

heart pumps. The vascular system, consisting of a vast network of

_____ , arterioles, capillaries, venules, and _____ ,

carries blood throughout the body. It keeps the heart filled with blood and maintains

_____ .

You gotta have heart

The heart's great vessels include the inferior and superior _____ , the

_____ , the pulmonary artery, and four pulmonary veins. The heart is

surrounded by a thin sac known as the _____ . Four chambers—two

_____ and two _____ —divide the heart and help keep

blood flowing through specific pathways. The heart's _____ keep blood

flowing in only one direction.

And the beat goes on

Heart contractions occur in a rhythm known as the _____ . They're

regulated by impulses that normally begin at the _____ node, the

heart's pacemaker. _____ marks the period when the heart

contracts and sends blood on its outward journey, and _____

is the period when the heart relaxes and fills with blood.

Options
aorta
arteries
atria
autonomic
blood pressure
cardiac cycle
diastole
oxygenated
pericardium
sinoatrial
systole
valves
veins
venae cavae
ventricles
waste products

All major vessels are present and accounted for, Sir!

■ Match point

Match the anatomical heart structure in column 1 with its definition in column 2.

Heart structure

1. Semilunar valves _____
2. Left atrium _____
3. Inferior vena cava _____
4. Chordae tendineae _____
5. Right atrium _____
6. Coronary sinus _____
7. Aortic arch _____
8. Superior vena cava _____
9. Epicardium _____
10. Right ventricle _____
11. Atrioventricular valves _____
12. Interventricular septum _____
13. Left ventricle _____

Definition

A. Vessel that receives blood from the upper part of the body

B. Lower heart chamber that pumps blood through aorta and out to rest of the body

C. Fibrous tissues that anchor valve leaflets to the heart wall

D. Tricuspid and mitral valves

E. Vessel that returns blood from the myocardium back to the heart

F. Upper heart chamber that receives oxygenated blood from pulmonary veins

G. Wall separating the lower heart chambers

H. Pulmonic and aortic valves

I. Vessel that receives blood from the lower part of the body

J. Upper segment of aorta located between the ascending and descending portions

K. Upper heart chamber that receives deoxygenated blood

L. Lower heart chamber that ejects blood through the pulmonic valve and into the pulmonary artery and lungs for oxygenation

M. Inner pericardial layer

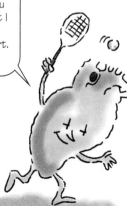

'Thirty love'... A lot of people think that the 'love' in tennis derives from the French word 'l'oeuf,' meaning 'egg' (you know, like a big goose egg), but I like to think that it had something to do with the heart. I'm such a romantic fellow!

■ Finish line

Identify the great vessels and heart chambers shown in the illustration below.

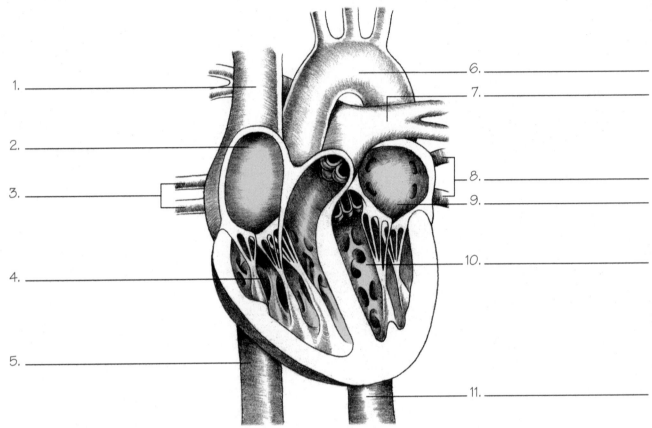

1. _____

2. _____

3. _____

4. _____

5. _____

6. _____

7. _____

8. _____

9. _____

10. _____

11. _____

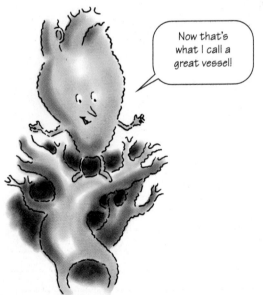

Now that's what I call a great vessel!

Team colors

Trace the path of blood flow through the heart, and color sections blue where deoxygenated blood flows and red where oxygenated blood flows.

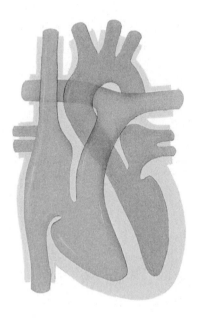

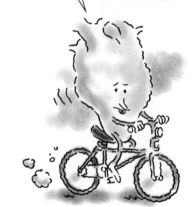

I wonder how many cycles I log on this thing each day... any guesses?

You make the call

Identify and briefly describe the steps of the cardiac cycle illustrated here.

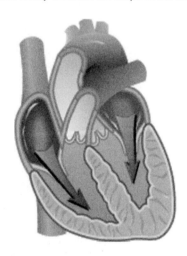

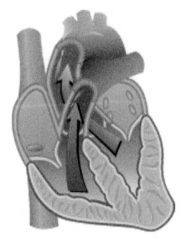

1. _____

_____

_____

_____

2. _____

_____

_____

_____

■ Match point

Match the heart sound in column 1 with its defining characteristics in column 2.

Heart sound

Defining characteristcs

1. S_1 _____
2. S_2 _____
3. S_3 _____
4. S_4 _____

A. Low-pitched galloping sound (similar to the y in "Ken-tuck-y") caused by rapid ventricular filling and best heard with patient lying on his left side

B. Low-pitched, dull "lub" sound that's best heard over the mitral area and caused by rising ventricular pressure and closure of the mitral and tricuspid valves at the beginning of systole

C. Adventitious sound called an *atrial gallop* (similar to the word "Ten-nes-see") that occurs when the atria contract and eject blood into resistant ventricles

D. Short, high-pitched "dub" sound best heard at the base of the heart at the end of systole, when ventricular pressure falls and aortic and pulmonic valves close

■ Brain crunches

Name nine arterial sites where peripheral pulses can be palpated.

1. _____
2. _____
3. _____
4. _____
5. _____
6. _____
7. _____
8. _____
9. _____

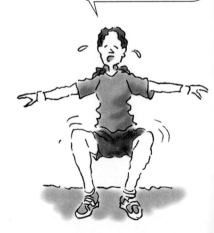

I said 'crunch time,' not 'brunch time'! Cruise people!

■ Hit or miss

Indicate whether the following statements about the vascular system are true or false.

_____ 1. Nearly all arteries carry oxygen-rich blood from the heart to the rest of the body.

_____ 2. The wall of an artery is thinner and more pliable than the wall of a vein.

_____ 3. Arteries contain valves at periodic intervals to prevent blood from flowing backward.

_____ 4. Capillaries are connected to arteries and veins through intermediary vessels called arterioles and venules.

_____ 5. The pulmonary vein is the only vein that carries oxygenated blood; all the rest carry deoxygenated blood.

_____ 6. The vascular system is constantly filled with about 10 L of circulating blood.

_____ 7. All vessels have pulsations that can be felt anywhere on the body.

_____ 8. The vascular system delivers oxygen, nutrients, and other substances to the body's cells and removes the waste products of cellular metabolism.

_____ 9. The exchange of fluid, nutrients, and metabolic wastes between blood and cells occurs in arteries.

_____ 10. Veins serve as a large reservoir for circulating blood.

> Another millimeter and I'll be perfect. (All right…I guess you could say I'm a little vein!)

■ Jumble gym

Unscramble the words below to identify some of the body's major arteries and veins. Then unscramble the circled letters to answer the question.

Question: **Which vessel returns blood from the lower part of the body to the heart?**

1. D I S S L A R O   S P I D E   _ _ _ _ _ _〇_   _〇_ _ _

2. A L R N U   _ _〇_ _

3. L A M E R O F 〇〇_ _ _ _ _

4. C H E R A B H A I L C I C O P   _〇_ _ _〇_ _ _ _ _ _〇_ _ _

5. S A I L V U N C A B   _ _ _ _ _ _〇_〇_

6. E N V S T E A R S R   I U S S N   _ _ _〇_〇_ _ _ _   _ _ _ _ _

7. N M O M C O   C I A I L 〇_ _ _〇_   _ _ _ _ _ _

8. T A R O A   _ _〇_〇

Answer: _ _ _ _ _ _ _ _   _ _ _ _   _ _ _ _

A-maze-ing race

Try not to skip a beat as you wind your way through this heart-pumping maze. If you enter through the superior vena cava and successfully exit through one of these vessels, you'll be rewarded with a breath of fresh air.
Name the vessel and the pathway.

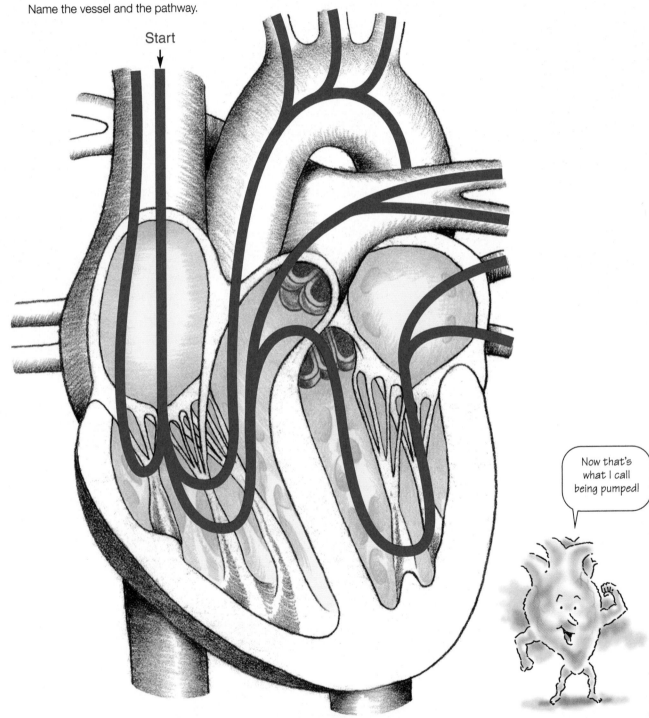

Start

Now that's what I call being pumped!

Team colors

Here's a game to really stretch your neurons! First identify the arteries and veins illustrated in this picture. Then circle with a colored pencil the nine sites where arterial pulses can be palpated. (Here's a hint: arteries are pictured in red, veins in gray.)

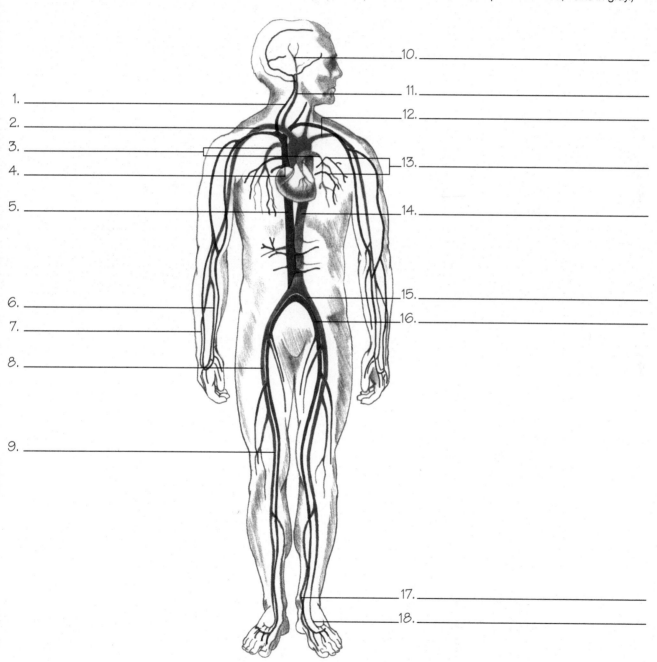

1. _____

2. _____

3. _____

4. _____

5. _____

6. _____

7. _____

8. _____

9. _____

10. _____

11. _____

12. _____

13. _____

14. _____

15. _____

16. _____

17. _____

18. _____

■ Brain crunches

Think fast…Can you identify at least 10 of the most commonly reported complaints given by patients with a cardiovascular problem?

1. _____
2. _____
3. _____
4. _____
5. _____
6. _____
7. _____
8. _____
9. _____
10. _____

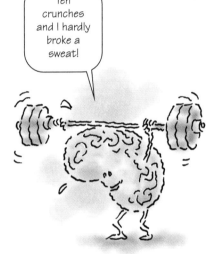

Ten crunches and I hardly broke a sweat!

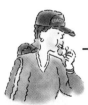

Coaching session
Age-related cardiovascular changes

Changes in the cardiovascular system occur as a natural part of the aging process. Unfortunately, these changes place elderly patients at higher risk for cardiovascular disorders than younger patients. During your assessment, keep in mind these age-related changes:

• slight decrease in heart size
• loss of cardiac contractile strength and efficiency
• decrease in cardiac output of 30% to 35% by age 70
• thickening of heart valves, causing incomplete valve closure (and systolic murmur)
• increase in left ventricular wall thickness of 25% between ages 30 and 80
• fibrous tissue infiltration of sinoatrial node and internodal atrial tracts, causing atrial fibrillation and flutter
• dilation and stretching of veins
• decline in coronary artery blood flow of 35% between ages 20 and 60
• increased aortic rigidity
• increased amount of time necessary for heart rate to return to normal after exercise
• decreased strength and elasticity of blood vessels, contributing to arterial and venous insufficiency
• decreased ability to respond to physical and emotional stress.

■■
■ Gear up!

Check off which equipment and supplies you'll need to conduct a cardiovascular assessment.

☐ Gloves
☐ Felt-tipped pen or marker
☐ Cotton-tipped applicators
☐ Stethoscope with bell and diaphragm
☐ Blood pressure cuff
☐ Measuring tape
☐ Ruler
☐ Povidone-iodine solution

☐ Penlight
☐ Otoscope
☐ Nasal speculum
☐ Tongue blade
☐ Tuning fork
☐ Syringes
☐ Needles
☐ Specimen containers

My secret to health, happiness, and longevity? That's easy...I follow a 13-step program every day and never take the elevator.

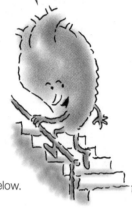

■■
■ Photo finish

Indicate the correct placement of these critical cardiovascular landmarks on the graphic photos below.

Anterior thorax view
- Epigastric area
- Sternoclavicular area
- Aortic area
- Xiphoid process
- Tricuspid (right ventricular) area
- Pulmonic area
- Midsternal line
- Midclavicular line
- Suprasternal notch
- Mitral (left ventricular) area

Lateral thorax view
- Midaxillary line
- Posterior axillary line
- Anterior axillary line

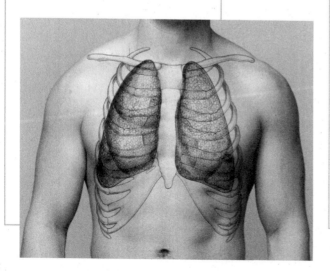

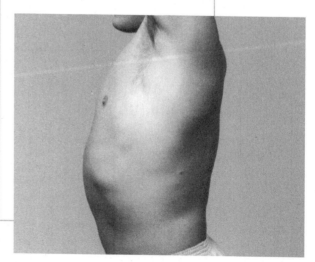

■ Choose the best course

Insert these steps in the boxes below to show the correct sequence for proceeding with a heart assessment.

Steps

Percuss heart to locate cardiac borders.

Inspect chest (note landmarks, pulsations, symmetry, retractions, heaves, and point of maximum impulse).

Auscultate for heart sounds, murmurs, and friction rubs.

Assess general appearance (body shape and size), skin (color, temperature, turgor, and texture), and alertness.

Palpate precordium to find apical impulse, noting thrills; also palpate sternoclavicular, aortic, pulmonic, tricuspid, and epigastric areas for abnormal pulsations.

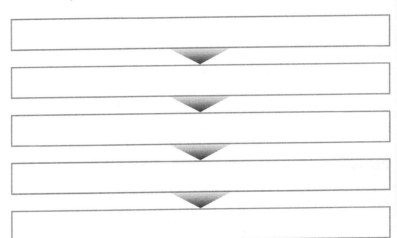

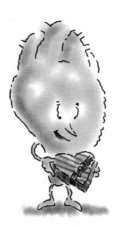

In case you need an extra box, I keep a few on hand for special occasions.

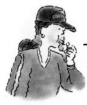

Coaching session
Finding and assessing the apical impulse

The apical impulse is associated with the first heart sound and carotid pulsation. To find the impulse and ensure that you aren't feeling a muscle spasm, use one hand to palpate the patient's carotid artery and the other to palpate the apical impulse. Then compare the timing and regularity of the impulses. The apical impulse should coincide roughly with the carotid pulsation.

Note the amplitude, size, intensity, location, and duration of the apical impulse. You should feel a gentle pulsation in an area about ½" to ¾" (1.5 to 2 cm) in diameter.

Pep talk

You can always amend a big plan, but you can never expand a little one. I don't believe in little plans. I believe in plans big enough to meet a situation which we can't possibly foresee now.

—Harry S Truman

■ ■
■ Hit or miss

Indicate whether the following statements about cardiac auscultation are true or false.

_____ 1. S_4 heart sounds are more common in elderly patients and those with hypertension, aortic stenosis, or a history of myocardial infarction.

_____ 2. Murmurs can be detected only during diastole.

_____ 3. The best way to hear aortic and pulmonic valve murmurs is with the patient lying on his left side.

_____ 4. A friction rub has a scratchy, rubbing quality.

_____ 5. Murmurs are commonly graded according to their intensity.

_____ 6. You can sometimes hear a split S_2 sound when the pulmonic valve closes later than the aortic valve during expiration.

_____ 7. The bell of the stethoscope is used to hear low-pitched sounds, and the diaphragm is used to hear high-pitched sounds.

_____ 8. S_3 sounds are a normal finding in children and are always considered abnormal after age 12.

_____ 9. Murmurs result when structural defects in the heart's chambers cause turbulent blood flow.

_____ 10. It's best to auscultate for heart sounds with the patient in three positions—lying on his back with the head of the bed raised 30 to 45 degrees, sitting up, and lying on his left side.

■ ■
■ Match point

Match the murmur grade in column 1 with its defining characteristics in column 2.

Murmur grade

1. Grade I _____
2. Grade II _____
3. Grade III _____
4. Grade IV _____
5. Grade V _____
6. Grade VI _____

Defining characteristics

A. Moderately loud, without a thrust or thrill

B. Loud enough to be heard before the stethoscope comes into contact with the chest

C. Barely audible murmur

D. Very loud, with a thrust or thrill

E. Audible but quiet and soft

F. Loud, with a thrill

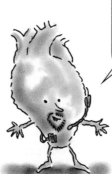

I was pretty impressed...I'd have to grade that murmur as a perfect "V," Ryan.

Pep talk

The way to happiness: keep your heart free from hate, your mind from worry. Live simply, expect little, give much. Fill your life with love. Scatter sunshine. Forget self, think of others. Do as you would be done by. Try this for a week and you will be surprised.

—Norman Vincent Peale

■ Step aerobics

Identify the position pictured in each photo, and explain briefly which sounds it's best suited to detect during auscultation.

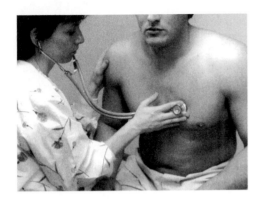

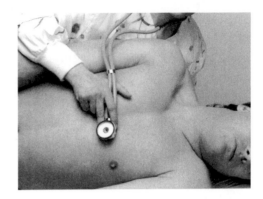

1. _____

_____

_____

2. _____

_____

_____

■ Team up!

Write each assessment finding under the appropriate heading to differentiate internal jugular vein pulsations from carotid artery pulsations.

Internal jugular vein pulsations

_____

_____

_____

_____

_____

Carotid artery pulsations

_____

_____

_____

_____

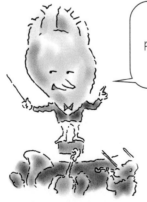

No, no!! I want to hear more pulsations, jugulars, with the second movement!

Assessment findings
- No decrease noted when patient is upright
- Soft, undulating pulsation
- Pulsation detected about 1½″ (4 cm) above sternal notch
- Pulsation changes in response to position
- No change noted when patient inhales
- Pulsation changes in response to breathing
- Pulsation detected just lateral to trachea and below jaw line
- Pulsation changes in response to palpation
- Brisk, localized pulsation
- No change noted with palpation

■ You make the call

Identify the arterial pulses being assessed in the pictures below.

1. _____

2. _____

3. _____

4. _____

5. _____

6. _____

7. _____

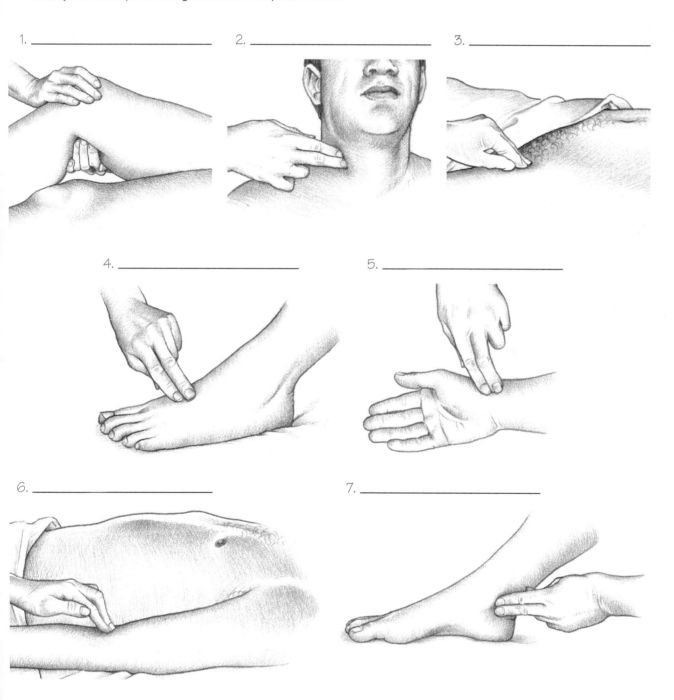

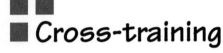 Cross-training

You've been working so hard...take a few minutes to relax, grab a smoothie, and de-stress with this crossword puzzle on cardiovascular abnormalities.

Across

2. Abnormal heart sounds caused by turbulent blood flow

5. Symptom commonly associated with an MI (two words)

6. Inability of heart to fill with or pump a sufficient amount of blood to body (two words)

9. Murmurlike sound of vascular, not cardiac, origin

10. Blood pressure that's consistently lower than normal

12. Heart rate faster than 100 beats/minute

13. Bulging portion of aorta caused by weakness in the arterial wall (two words)

15. Third heart sound that's often the cardinal sign of heart failure in adults (two words)

17. Conscious awareness of one's heartbeat

Down

1. Heart attack, caused by interruption of the blood supply to the heart (two words)

3. Open sore on skin (commonly on feet or ankles) due to arterial or venous insufficiency

4. Abnormal cardiac waveform

7. Fourth heart sound commonly heard in those with hypertension (two words)

8. Bluish discoloration indicating poor cardiac output

11. Abnormally slow heart rate

14. Excessive tiredness, lack of energy, or exhaustion

16. Swelling that's often a sign of heart failure or venous insufficiency

■ Strikeout

Cross out the symptom that doesn't belong with each group of cardiovascular-related findings, and then identify the probable cause.

1. Sudden chest pain, lasting 30 minutes to 2 hours; shortness of breath; diaphoresis; weakness; anxiety; hearing loss:

_____

2. Moderate to severe bilateral leg edema, visual halos, darkened skin, stasis ulcers around the ankles:

_____

3. Paroxysmal or sustained palpitations; dizziness, weakness, and fatigue; stomach pain; irregular, rapid, or slow pulse rate; decreased blood pressure; confusion:

_____

4. Feeling of euphoria; aching, squeezing, heavy pressure; burning pain that usually subsides within 10 minutes:

_____

5. Sudden excruciating, tearing chest pain; pain radiating to back, neck, and shoulders; Grade VI murmur; blood pressure difference between right and left arm:

_____

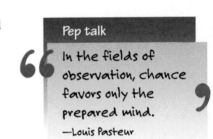

Pep talk

" In the fields of observation, chance favors only the prepared mind. "

—Louis Pasteur

■ Mind sprints

Explore which chest pain–related questions would be appropriate to ask your patient during a health assessment. Time yourself, and see how many questions you can list in 5 minutes.

_____
_____
_____
_____
_____
_____
_____
_____

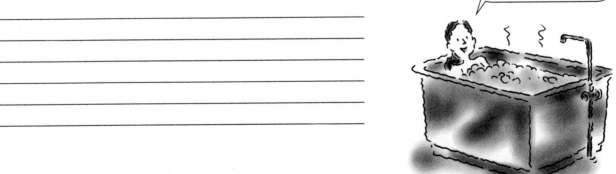

Keep plugging away. You're nearing the end of the chapter and maybe even a rewarding bubble bath—or whatever else floats your boat!

■ In the ballpark

Edema and pulses are both graded using a four-point scale. Fill in the missing information in the scales below to show how you would grade your patient's findings.

Edema grading scale	
+1	Finger leaves slight imprint (2-mm indentation)
+2	_____
+3	_____
+4	Finger leaves deep imprint that only slowly returns to normal (8-mm indentation)

Pulses grading scale	
4+	Bounding
3+	_____
2+	_____
1+	_____
0	Absent

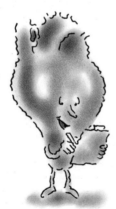

In case you were wondering...No, this game isn't being graded on a curve!

■ Winner's circle

Circle the illustration that best depicts chronic venous insufficiency.

1.

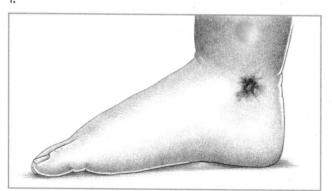

2.

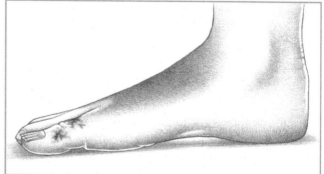

■ Match point

Determining whether your patient's chest pain is cardiac related can be a bit tricky. Let's see if you're up for the challenge. Match the assessment findings in column 1 with the probable cause in column 2.

Assessment findings

1. Sudden, stabbing pain over the lung area; may be accompanied by cyanosis, dyspnea, or cough with hemoptysis _____

2. Sharp, continuous substernal pain that can radiate to the neck or left arm; occurs suddenly and may be accompanied by friction rub _____

3. Dull, pressurelike, squeezing pain in the substernal and epigastric areas _____

4. Burning feeling in epigastric area that occurs after eating; sometimes accompanied by hematemesis or tarry stools and usually subsides within 20 minutes _____

5. Continuous or intermittent sharp pain that occurs anywhere in the chest; may occur gradually or suddenly and can be tender to the touch _____

6. Sudden tightness or pressure across the chest (sometimes radiating to the jaw, neck, arms, or back) that lasts 30 minutes to 2 hours; may be accompanied by shortness of breath, diaphoresis, weakness, anxiety, or nausea _____

7. Sharp, severe pain over the lower chest or upper abdomen _____

8. Sudden dull or stabbing pain occurring anywhere in the chest that's usually accompanied by hyperventilation or breathlessness; may last less than 1 minute or up to several days _____

Probable cause

A. Acute myocardial infarction

B. Esophageal spasm

C. Peptic ulcer

D. Acute anxiety

E. Pulmonary embolus

F. Hiatal hernia

G. Pericarditis

H. Chest-wall syndrome

Winded, sweaty, tired, and a little achy matches up with one good cardiovascular workout in my book.

Train your brain

Sound out each group of pictures and symbols to reveal terms that complete this assessment consideration.

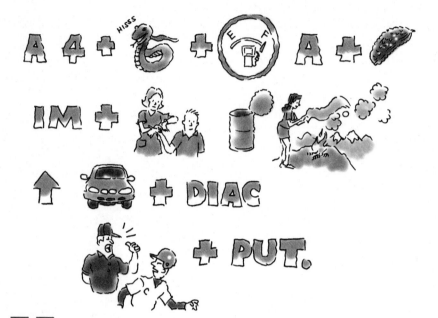

Batter's box

Fill in the blanks wth the correct words and you'll have a handy list of important facts about abnormal pulsations.

- A displaced apical impulse may indicate an enlarged _____ ,
1

which may be caused by heart failure or hypertension.

- Pulsations in the aortic, pulmonic, or tricuspid areas may signal an

enlarged _____ or _____ disease.
2   3

- Increased cardiac output or an aortic aneurysm may produce pulsations

in the _____ area.
4

- A pulsation in the sternoclavicular area suggests an _____ .
5

- A _____ is a palpable vibration that usually suggests
6

valvular dysfunction.

Options
aortic

aortic aneurysm

heart chamber

left ventricle

thrill

valvular

You make the call

Identify the abnormal arterial pulses based on the descriptions and accompanying waveforms.

1. Has a regular, alternating pattern of a weak and a strong pulse; associated with left-sided heart failure:

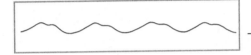

_____

2. Has a decreased amplitude with a slower upstroke and downstroke; causes include increased peripheral vascular resistance and decreased stroke volume:

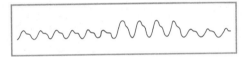

_____

3. Has increases and decreases in amplitude associated with the respiratory cycle; associated with pericardial tamponade, advanced heart failure, and constrictive pericarditis:

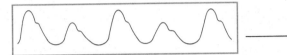

_____

4. Shows an initial upstroke, a subsequent downstroke, then another upstroke during systole; caused by aortic stenosis and aortic insufficiency:

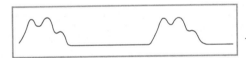

_____

5. Has a sharp upstroke and downstroke with a pointed peak, and the amplitude is elevated; causes include increased stroke volume or stiffness of arterial walls:

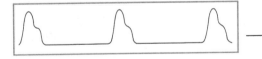

_____

6. Has an irregular, alternating pattern of a weak and a strong pulse; caused by premature atrial or ventricular beats:

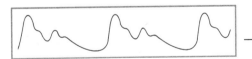

_____

Brain crunches

Here's a two-part exercise—simply to test your knowledge of cardiovascular assessment and increase your pulse rate.

As quickly as you can, list seven lifestyle and environmental factors that can affect your patient's cardiovascular health.

1. _____
2. _____
3. _____
4. _____
5. _____
6. _____
7. _____

Now, list six criteria commonly used to describe murmurs.

1. _____
2. _____
3. _____
4. _____
5. _____
6. _____

Three-point conversion

Identify the cardiovascular symptoms best depicted in the illustrations below.

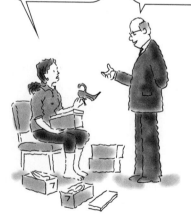

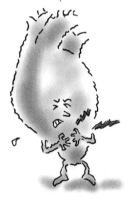

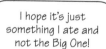

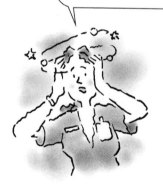

1. _____ 2. _____ 3. _____

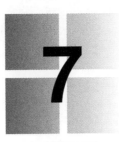

7

Respiratory system

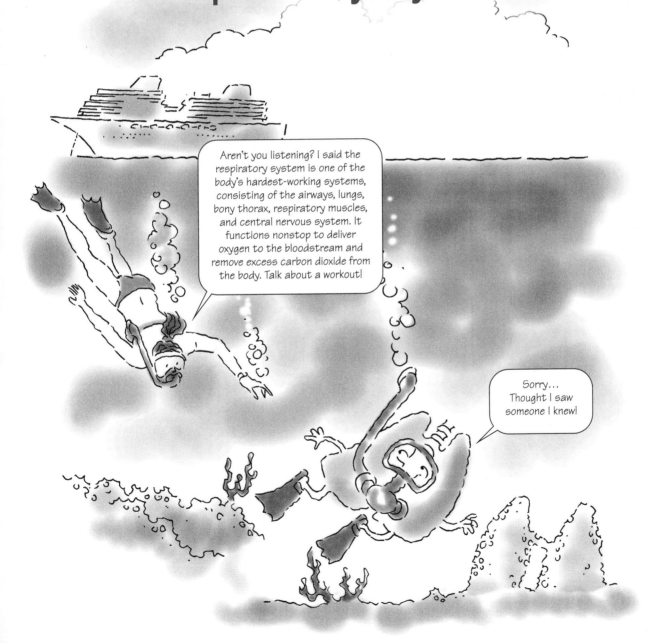

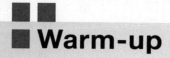
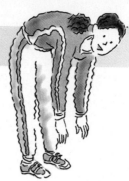

Warm-up

Respiratory system review

Structures and functions

Upper airways

- Include the nasopharynx, oropharynx, laryngopharynx, and larynx
- Warm, filter, and humidify inhaled air
- Help to make sound and send air to lower airways

Lower airways

- Trachea—divides into the right and left mainstem bronchi and continues to divide into smaller passages
- Bronchioles—terminate in the alveolar ducts and the alveoli
- Alveoli—gas-exchanging units of the lungs

Thorax

- Includes the clavicles, sternum, scapulae, 12 sets of ribs (which allow the chest to expand and contract during each breath), and 12 thoracic vertebrae

Respiratory muscles

- Diaphragm and external intercostal muscles (primary breathing muscles)—contract on inhalation and relax on exhalation
- Accessory inspiratory muscles (trapezius, sternocleidomastoid, and scalenes)—combine to elevate the scapulae, clavicle, sternum, and upper ribs when primary breathing muscles aren't effective

Health history

- Ask patient about shortness of breath, and rate his dyspnea on a scale of 0 to 10.
- Determine if patient has orthopnea, and ask how many pillows he uses to sleep at night.
- Ask if patient has a cough. If he does, ask him if it's productive or nonproductive. If it's productive, have him describe the sputum.
- Have patient describe any chest pain, including its location, how it feels, if it radiates, what causes it, and what makes it feel better.
- Ask about the patient's medical history, including smoking, pneumonia, and exposure to irritants.

Assessment

Inspection

- Watch for chest-wall symmetry as the patient breathes. Note any paradoxical, or uneven, chest-wall movement.
- Count patient's respiratory rate for a full minute (longer if you note abnormalities); normal respiratory rate for an adult is 12 to 20 breaths/minute; up to 40 breaths/minute for infants.
- Observe patient's respiratory pattern; it should be even, coordinated, and regular with occasional sighs.
- Inspect the skin, tongue, mouth, fingers, and nail beds, which can provide more information about the patient's respiratory status.

Palpation

- Gently use your palms to palpate the chest for crepitus, tenderness, alignment, bulging, or retractions. Palpate the front and back of the chest.
- Use the pads of your fingers to palpate the chest, including over the ribs. Note skin temperature, turgor, and moisture as well as the presence of scars, lumps, lesions, or ulcerations.
- Palpate for tactile fremitus.
- Assess chest-wall symmetry and expansion by placing your hands on the front of the chest with thumbs touching each other, and ask the patient to inhale deeply.

Percussion

- Resonant sounds are heard over normal lung tissue.
- Hyperresonance is found over areas of increased air in the lung or pleural space (hyperinflated lung, emphysema).
- Dullness is found over areas of decreased air in the lungs (atelectasis, pneumonia).
- Flatness is found over consolidated areas (atelectasis, pleural effusion).
- Tympany is found over areas where air has collected (large pneumothorax).

Auscultation

- Use the diaphragm of the stethoscope to listen to a full inspiration and a full expiration at each site.
- Ask patient to breathe through his mouth. (Nose breathing alters the pitch of breath sounds.)
- Wet chest hair to prevent crackles that would be heard if auscultating over dry hair.

NORMAL BREATH SOUNDS

- Tracheal—harsh, high-pitched, and discontinuous
- Bronchial—loud, high-pitched, and discontinuous
- Bronchovesicular—medium-pitched and continuous
- Vesicular—soft and low-pitched

VOCAL FREMITUS

- Bronchophony—ask the patient to say "ninety-nine"
- Egophony—ask the patient to say "E"
- Whispered pectoriloquy—ask the patient to whisper "1, 2, 3"

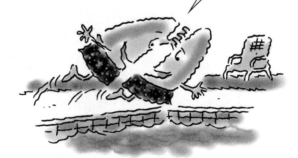

Did you know that wetting your patient's chest hair before auscultation will prevent you from hearing crackles caused by dry hair?

Abnormal findings

Chest-wall abnormalities

- Barrel chest—large front-to-back diameter
- Pigeon chest—sternum protrudes beyond front of abdomen; increased front-to-back diameter of chest
- Funnel chest—depression on all or part of the sternum
- Thoracic kyphoscoliosis—curvature of spine; rotation of vertebrae; distortion of lung tissues

Abnormal respiratory patterns

- Tachypnea—respiratory rate greater than 20 breaths/minute with shallow breathing
- Bradypnea—respiratory rate below 10 breaths/minute
- Apnea—the absence of breathing; may be life-threatening if it lasts long
- Hyperpnea—deep, rapid breathing
- Kussmaul's respirations—rapid, deep, sighing breaths
- Cheyne-Stokes respirations—deep breaths alternating with periods of apnea
- Biot's respirations—rapid, deep breaths that alternate with abrupt apneic periods

Abnormal breath sounds

- Crackles—intermittent, nonmusical, crackling sounds heard during inspiration; classified as fine or coarse
- Wheezes—high-pitched sounds caused by blocked airflow, heard on exhalation
- Rhonchi—low-pitched snoring or rattling sound; heard primarily on exhalation
- Stridor—loud, high-pitched sound heard during inspiration
- Pleural friction rub—low-pitched grating sound heard during inspiration and expiration; accompanied by pain

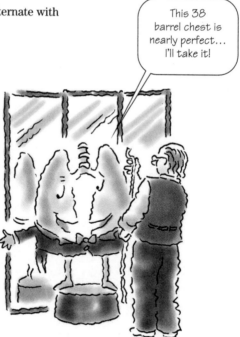

■ Finish line

Identify the major structures of the respiratory system shown in this illustration.

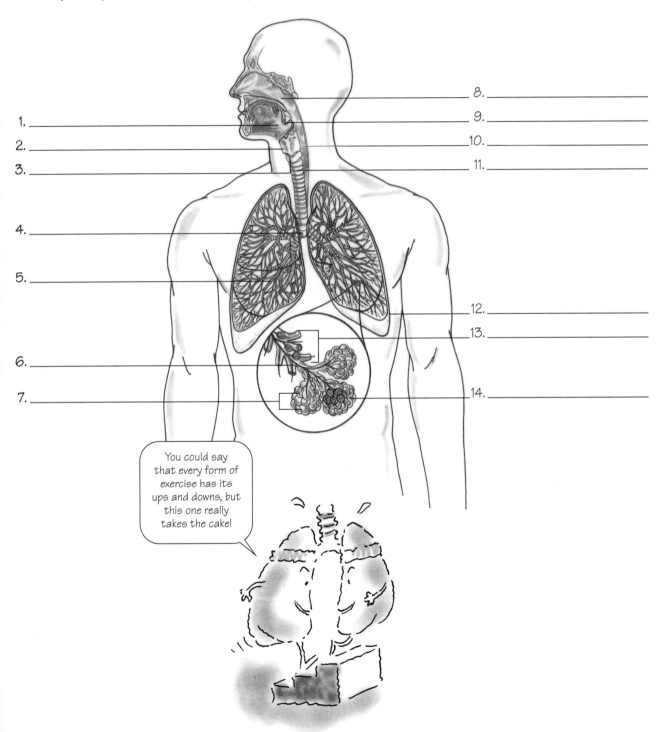

1. _____

2. _____

3. _____

4. _____

5. _____

6. _____

7. _____

8. _____

9. _____

10. _____

11. _____

12. _____

13. _____

14. _____

You could say that every form of exercise has its ups and downs, but this one really takes the cake!

■■
■ Hit or miss

Indicate whether the following statements about the respiratory system are true or false.

_____ 1. The epiglottis is a hard, bonelike structure that closes the bottom of the larynx when the patient swallows, protecting him from aspirating food and fluid into the lower airways.

_____ 2. The larynx houses the vocal cords and serves as the transition point between the upper and lower airways.

_____ 3. The left lung is smaller than the right lung and has only two lobes.

_____ 4. All areas that come in contact with the lungs in the thoracic cavity are lined with visceral pleura.

_____ 5. The eighth, ninth, and tenth ribs attach to the cartilage of the preceding rib as well as to the thoracic vertebrae.

_____ 6. The diaphragm and external intercostal muscles relax when a patient inhales and contract when he exhales.

_____ 7. Accessory inspiratory muscles include the trapezius, the sternocleidomastoid, and the scalenes.

_____ 8. If a patient has an airway obstruction, he may use the abdominal muscles and internal intercostal muscles to exhale.

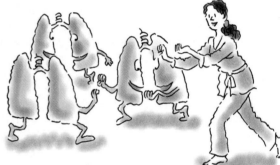

Breathe correctly and find your chi, Grasshoppers!

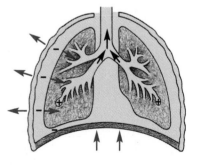

■■
■ You make the call

Identify and briefly explain the breathing mechanisms occurring in each of the illustrations below.

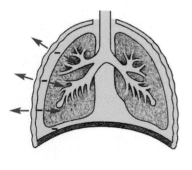

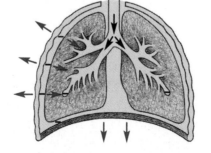

1. _____

_____

_____

_____

_____

2. _____

_____

_____

_____

_____

3. _____

_____

_____

_____

_____

■ Finish line

Identify the common landmarks used in a respiratory assessment in each of the illustrations below.

Anterior view

1. _____
2. _____
3. _____
4. _____
5. _____

6. _____
7. _____

8. _____
9. _____
10. _____
11. _____

12. _____
13. _____
14. _____
15. _____

Posterior view

1. _____
2. _____
3. _____

4. _____

5. _____

6. _____

7. _____
8. _____

9. _____

10. _____

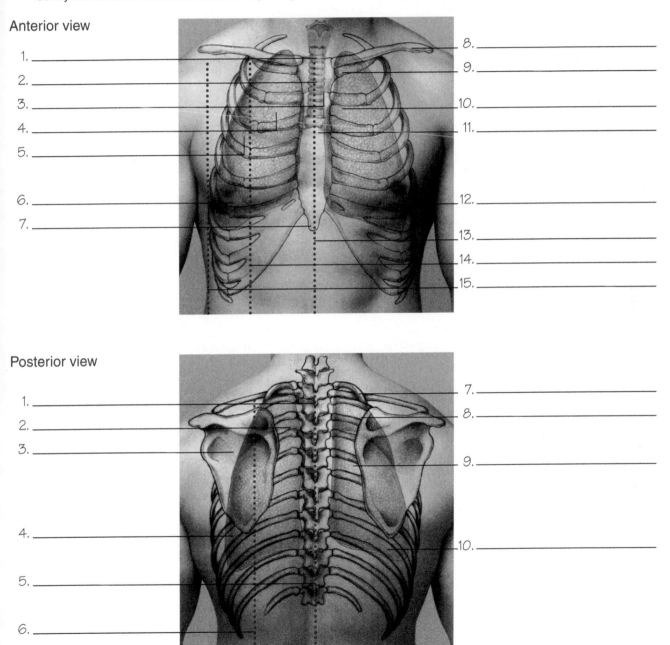

■ Brain crunches

Take a quick breath, then fire away! Name six common respiratory complaints identified by patients with a respiratory condition during a health history.

1. _____
2. _____
3. _____
4. _____
5. _____
6. _____

■ Winner's circle

Circle the illustration that best shows a need for further patient teaching about respiratory problems.

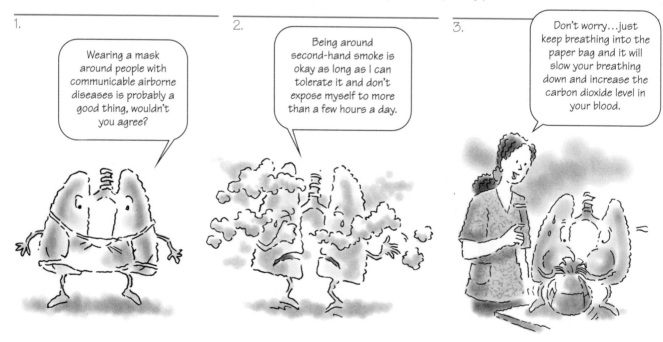

1. Wearing a mask around people with communicable airborne diseases is probably a good thing, wouldn't you agree?

2. Being around second-hand smoke is okay as long as I can tolerate it and don't expose myself to more than a few hours a day.

3. Don't worry...just keep breathing into the paper bag and it will slow your breathing down and increase the carbon dioxide level in your blood.

Mind sprints

Go the distance by listing which assessment questions you should ask your patient about his cough.
Time yourself, and see how many questions you can list in 5 minutes.

_____

_____

_____

_____

_____

_____

_____

_____

_____

_____

> What...I'm pacing myself!

Coaching session
Grading dyspnea

You can obtain a history of your patient's shortness of breath by using several scales. To assess dyspnea as objectively as possible, ask him to briefly describe how various activities affect his breathing. Then document his response using this grading system:

Grade 0: not troubled by breathlessness except with strenuous exercise

Grade 1: troubled by shortness of breath when hurrying on a level path or walking up a slight hill

Grade 2: walks more slowly on a level path than people of the same age because of breathlessness, or has to stop to breathe when walking on a level path at his own pace

Grade 3: stops to breathe after walking about 100 yards (91 m) on a level path

Grade 4: too breathless to leave the house, or breathless when dressing or undressing

Match point

Match the respiratory assessment term in column 1 with its corresponding definition in column 2.

Respiratory assessment term

1. Paradoxical breathing _____
2. Cyanosis _____
3. Crepitus _____
4. Tactile fremitus _____
5. Bronchovesicular _____
6. Crackles _____
7. Pursed-lip breathing _____
8. Hyperpnea _____
9. Whispered pectoriloquy _____
10. Atelectasis _____

Definition

A. Abnormal breath sounds caused by fluid in the airways

B. Bluish tint to skin, mucous membranes, and nail beds that's a late sign of hypoxemia

C. Transmitted voice sound heard during auscultation that occurs over consolidated areas

D. Grating, crackling, or popping sounds and sensations detected during palpation that indicate subcutaneous air in the chest

E. Collapse of all or part of the lung

F. Uneven movement of the chest wall indicating loss of chest wall function

G. Palpable vibrations caused by transmission of air through the bronchopulmonary system

H. Deep, fast breathing

I. Breathing technique that prolongs exhalation to slow the breathing rate

J. Normal, medium-loud breath sound heard continuously when patient inhales or exhales

Keep plugging away...we're all rooting for you!

Step aerobics

Use arrows to show the correct pattern or sequence you'd follow when assessing normal and abnormal breath sounds during percussion and auscultation.

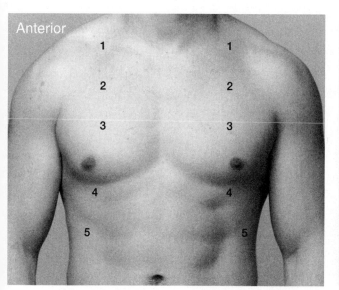

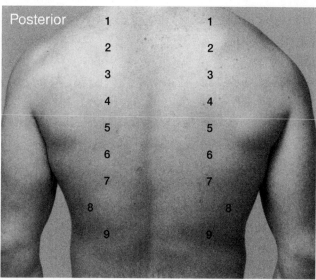

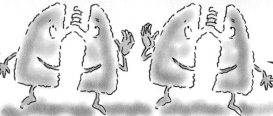

> Remember, you need to listen to both sides of your patient's chest.

> That's right...and always follow the same sequence.

You make the call

Complete this chart to test your skill at differentiating percussion sounds and identifying their clinical significance.

Sound	Description	Clinical significance
Flat	Short, soft, high-pitched, extremely dull sound	Consolidation, as in atelectasis and extensive pleural effusion
Dull	_____	Solid area, as in lobar pneumonia
Resonant	Long, loud, low-pitched, hollow sound	_____
Hyperresonant	Very loud, lower-pitched sound	_____
Tympanic	_____	Air collection, as in gastric bubbles or large pneumothorax

Match point

Listen up…this one's really easy. Match the normal breath sound in column 1 with its descriptive quality in column 2.

Normal breath sound

1. Vesicular _____
2. Bronchial _____
3. Tracheal _____
4. Bronchovesicular _____

Descriptive quality

A. Medium in loudness and pitch
B. Loud, high-pitched
C. Soft, low-pitched
D. Harsh, high-pitched

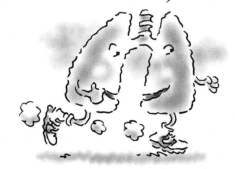

After this lap, the next sound you hear from me will be a sigh of relief!

Photo finish

Now use these diagrams to show where you'd expect to auscultate the normal breath sounds identified in the previous game.

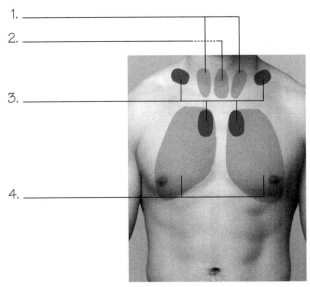

1. _____
2. _____
3. _____
4. _____

Anterior thorax

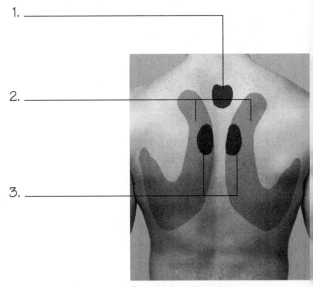

1. _____
2. _____
3. _____

Posterior thorax

■ Team up!

One or both lungs? Where you hear diminished but normal breath sounds may point to a specific type of respiratory problem. Write the potential problem under the appropriate heading.

One lung

_____

_____

_____

_____

_____

Both lungs

_____

_____

_____

_____

_____

Potential problems
- Pleural effusion
- Atelectasis
- Severe bronchospasm
- Pneumothorax
- Emphysema
- Tumor
- Mucus plugs in airways
- Shallow breathing

Pep talk

To live is not merely to breathe:
It is to act; it is to make use of
our organs, senses, faculties—of
all those parts of ourselves
which give us feeling of
existence.

—Jean Jacques Rousseau

■ You make the call

Identify the assessment technique shown in each photo and tell briefly why it's used.

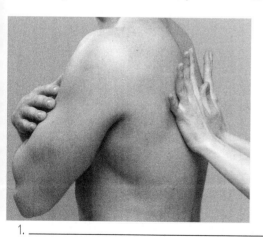

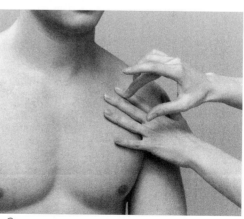

1. _____

_____

_____

_____

2. _____

_____

_____

_____

Choose the best course

Put these steps in the correct order to show how you would measure the distance your patient's diaphragm moves during inspiration and expiration. Then answer this question: What's the normal distance the diaphragm moves?

Steps

Use a pen to mark diaphragm's position at full inspiration.

Ask patient to exhale.

Use a pen to mark diaphragm's position at full expiration.

Percuss the back to locate diaphragm after patient breathes in fully.

Repeat procedure on opposite side of back.

Percuss the back on one side to locate the upper edge of diaphragm.

Use a ruler or tape measure to determine distance between marks.

Ask patient to inhale as deeply as possible.

Answer: _____

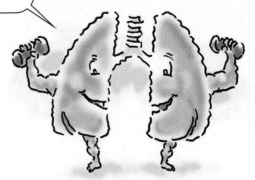

Here's an interesting fact...Men, children, infants, athletes, and singers typically use diaphragmatic (abdominal) breathing, whereas most women use intercostal (chest) breathing.

I love going for extra points!

Three-point conversion

Asking your patient to repeat certain words during auscultation can help you assess for vocal fremitus. Identify which abnormal voice sounds (bronchophony, egophony, whispered pectoriloquy) are characterized in the illustrations below. For extra points, tell how the sounds would differ over normal and consolidated lung tissue.

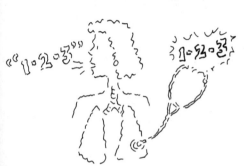

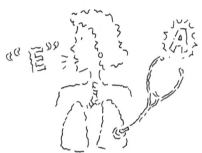

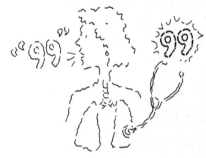

1. _____

2. _____

3. _____

Strikeout

Here's one way to take off some excess weight in a hurry…Trim these oversized statements by crossing out the assessment term or phrase that doesn't belong.

1. Tactile fremitus is decreased over areas where pleural fluid collects, at times when the patient speaks softly, over large bronchial tubes, and in those with pneumothorax.

2. When palpating the chest wall, it should feel smooth, warm, rigid, and dry.

3. Inspection of the skin, mouth, tongue, fingers, toes, and nail beds may provide information about a patient's respiratory status.

4. Accessory inspiratory muscles include the trapezius, the sternocleidomastoid, the diaphragm, and the scalenes.

5. Chest pain associated with a respiratory problem usually results from asthma, pneumonia, pulmonary embolism, or pleural inflammation.

Match point

Take a long, deep breath before tackling this test. Match the pulmonary function test in column 1 with its corresponding definition in column 2.

Pulmonary function test

1. Vital capacity _____
2. Minute volume _____
3. Tidal volume _____
4. Expiratory reserve volume _____
5. Inspiratory reserve volume _____
6. Inspiratory capacity _____

Definition

A. Amount of air breathed per minute

B. Amount of air that can be inhaled after normal expiration

C. Amount of air inhaled or exhaled during normal breathing

D. Amount of air that can be exhaled after maximum inspiration

E. Amount of air that can be exhaled after normal expiration

F. Amount of air inhaled after normal inspiration

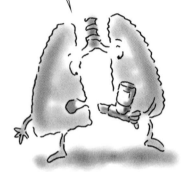

I'd offer you a puff, but sharing medications isn't medically recommended.

Train your brain

Sound out the pictures and symbols to reveal an important respiratory assessment tip.

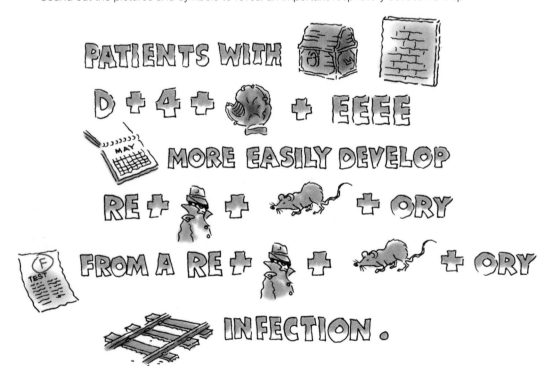

PATIENTS WITH [chest] [brick wall]

D + 4 + [elephant] + EEEE

[MAY calendar] MORE EASILY DEVELOP

RE + [spy] + [rat] + ORY

[F TEST] FROM A RE + [spy] + [rat] + ORY

[railroad track] INFECTION.

Answer: _____

Cross-training

Here's an exercise to stretch your knowledge of respiratory abnormalities.

Across

1. Lung condition resulting in inflamed, fluid-filled alveoli
6. Partial or complete lung collapse
9. Expectorated lung secretions
10. Abnormal sounds heard when collapsed or fluid-filled alveoli pop open
11. Shortness of breath
12. Bluish tint associated with reduced oxygen flow

Down

1. Air bubble in lung
2. Often requires use of an inhaler
3. Indication of subcutaneous air in chest
4. Low-pitched, snoring, rattling sounds
5. Shallow breathing occurring with an increased respiratory rate
7. High-pitched sounds that occur when airflow is blocked
8. Absence of breathing
10. Emphysema or chronic bronchitis (abbreviation)

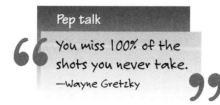

Pep talk

You miss 100% of the shots you never take.
—Wayne Gretzky

■ Match point

Match each of the chest deformities listed with the image that best depicts it.

1. _____   2. _____   3. _____   4. _____

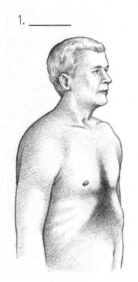
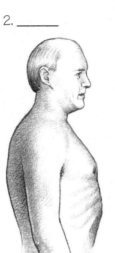
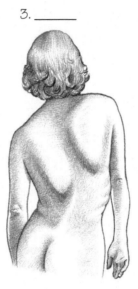
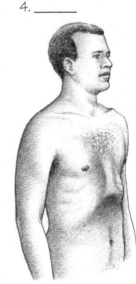

Chest deformity

A. Thoracic kyphoscoliosis

B. Pigeon chest

C. Funnel chest

D. Barrel chest

■ Hit or miss

Indicate whether the following statements about chest-wall abnormalities are true or false.

_____ 1. Chest-wall abnormalities may be congenital or acquired.

_____ 2. Chest-wall deformities always result in abnormal lung development.

_____ 3. Barrel chest can be normal in infants and elderly patients.

_____ 4. In patients with chronic obstructive pulmonary disease, a barrel chest indicates that lungs have lost their elasticity and that the diaphragm is raised.

_____ 5. Pectus excavatum is the other name for pigeon chest.

_____ 6. In thoracic kyphoscoliosis, the patient's spine curves to one side and the vertebrae are rotated.

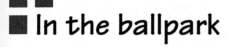

Let's see if I can sneak a curve ball or two by them!

■■ ■ In the ballpark

Match the level or measurement in column 1 with the normal adult respiratory finding in column 2.

Level or measurement

1. 300 million _____

2. < 90 _____

3. 1¼″ to 2″ (3 to 5 cm) _____

4. 12 to 20 _____

5. 1:2 _____

6. < 180 _____

7. 3″ (7.6 cm) _____

Normal adult respiratory finding

A. Respiratory rate (breaths/minute)

B. Inspiration to expiration ratio

C. Costal angle (degrees)

D. Nail bed angle (degrees)

E. Number of alveoli in lungs

F. Depth of structures assessed by percussion

G. Distance the diaphragm descends during inhalation

■■ ■ Brain crunches

Think fast…your patient's life may depend on your knowing the answer to this one!

Question: **What are eight respiratory-related signs and symptoms of airway obstruction?**

1. _____

2. _____

3. _____

4. _____

5. _____

6. _____

7. _____

8. _____

Jumble gym

Unscramble the words below to discover terms related to abnormal respiratory patterns.
Then use the circled letters to answer the question.

Question: What type of respiration has a regular pattern of variations in the rate and depth of breathing, with deep breaths alternating with short periods of apnea?

1. M U S K L A S U ◯ _ ◯◯ _ _ _ _

2. O T I B _ _ ◯◯

3. B E A D Y P R A N _ _ _ _ ◯ _ _ ◯ _

4. P R A Y H E E P N ◯ _ _ _ _ _ _ ◯ _

5. A P E C H A T N Y _ _ ◯ _ _ _ ◯ _ _

6. N A P A E _ _ _ ◯ _

Answer: _ _ _ _ _ _ - _ _ _ _ _

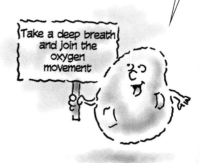

You can do it...only a few more exercises and you're on to the next chapter!

Take a deep breath and join the oxygen movement

Team up!

Insert the respiratory disorders boxed below under their most commonly associated sign or symptom.

Cough
_____
_____
_____
_____
_____
_____
_____

Dyspnea
_____
_____
_____
_____
_____
_____
_____

Hemoptysis
_____
_____
_____
_____
_____
_____

Wheezing
_____
_____
_____
_____
_____
_____

Respiratory disorders
- Acute respiratory distress syndrome
- Aspiration of a foreign body
- Asthma
- Atelectasis
- Chronic bronchitis
- Emphysema
- Lung cancer
- Pleural effusion
- Pneumonia
- Pulmonary edema
- Pulmonary embolism
- Pulmonary tuberculosis

■ You make the call

Identify the abnormal respiratory patterns shown here.

1. _____

2. _____

3. _____

4. _____

5. _____

6. _____

7. _____

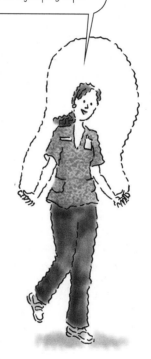

There's something about respiratory patterns that reminds me of a jumping rope!

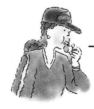

Coaching session

What to do when wheezing stops

If you no longer hear wheezing in a patient having an acute asthma attack, the attack may be far from over. When bronchospasm and mucosal swelling become severe, little air can move through the airways. As a result, you won't hear wheezing.

If all other assessment criteria—labored breathing, prolonged expiratory time, and accessory muscle use—point to acute bronchial obstruction, act to maintain the patient's airway and give oxygen as ordered. The patient may begin to wheeze again when the airways open.

■ Brain crunches

Bet you can answer this one in one deep breath…

Question: Can you identify five breath sounds that are considered adventitious?

1. _____
2. _____
3. _____
4. _____
5. _____

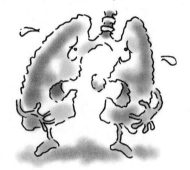

Give me a second or two and I'll help you out with that question…I'm having an adventitious moment!

■ Hit or miss

Identify whether the following statements about abnormal breath sounds are true or false.

_____ 1. Crackles are normally heard when the patient exhales, and they usually don't clear with coughing.

_____ 2. Pleural friction rub is a low-pitched, grating, rubbing sound caused when lung layers rub together.

_____ 3. Rhonchi usually change or disappear with coughing.

_____ 4. Fine crackles are also referred to as the "death rattle."

_____ 5. Loud, high-pitched crowing sounds (stridor) aren't usually a serious concern.

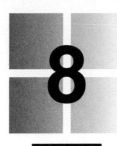

8

Breasts and axillae

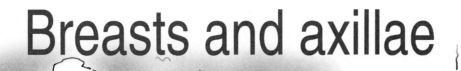

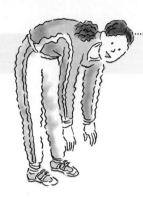

■■ **Warm-up**

Breasts and axillae review

Structures

■ Nipple—pigmented erectile tissue located in the center of each breast
■ Areola—ringed area that surrounds the nipple; darker in color than adjacent tissue
■ Cooper's ligaments—fibrous bands that support each breast
■ Glandular lobes—contain the alveoli that produce milk
■ Lactiferous ducts—transport milk from each lobe to the nipple

Health history

■ Ask patient about a history of breast lumps, breast surgery, breast cancer, fibrocystic breast disease, or other breast disorders.
■ Ask about the patient's menstrual and pregnancy history.
■ Ask about a family history of breast disorders, especially breast cancer.

Assessment

■ Inspect the breast, noting breast size and symmetry and skin condition.
■ Palpate each breast in concentric circles outward from the nipple, including the periphery, tail of Spence, and areola.
■ Palpate the nipple and compress to check for discharge.
■ Inspect and palpate the axilla.
■ Palpate lymph node chains.

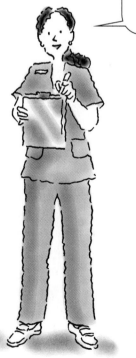

Remember to ask about your patient's menstrual and pregnancy history—both are pertinent to the breast and axillae evaluation.

Documenting a breast mass

Note these characteristics:

- Diameter
- Shape
- Consistency
- Mobility
- Degree of tenderness
- Location

Abnormal findings

- Breast nodule—breast lump that may be benign or malignant
- Breast dimpling—the puckering or retraction of skin on the breast
- Peau d'orange (orange peel skin)—the edematous thickening and pitting of breast skin
- Nipple retraction—inward displacement of the nipple below the level of surrounding breast tissue
- Nipple discharge—may be a normal finding or can signal serious disease
- Pain—may occur during rest or movement; may be aggravated by manipulation or palpation
- Visible veins—may indicate cancer but also occur normally in pregnant women

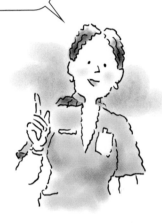

No matter how informed a woman is, she can still feel anxious during breast examinations, even if she hasn't noticed a problem. Keep in mind that the breast is more than just a delicate structure; it's a delicate subject.

■ ■
■ Batter's box

In this first exercise, we'll test your recall of vital statistics and important facts about breast anatomy and physiology. Fill in the blanks with the appropriate words and you'll have a handy checklist to tuck into your lab coat pocket.

1. Also called _____ glands, the breasts lie on the anterior chest wall.

2. The breasts are located vertically between the second or third and the sixth or seventh

ribs over the _____ muscle and the _____ muscle,

and horizontally between the sternal border and _____ line.

3. Each breast has a centrally located _____ ringed by an _____

that's darker than the adjacent tissue.

4. Sebaceous glands, also called _____ , are scattered on the areola surface.

5. Three types of tissues — _____ , _____ , and

_____ — support the breasts beneath the skin.

6. In women, the _____ ducts from each of the 12 to 25 glandular lobes

surrounding each breast transport milk to the nipple.

7. The breasts also hold several lymph node chains that drain _____ from

various areas of the chest, axilla, and upper arm.

8. In both men and women, the lymphatic system is the most common route of spread of

cells that cause _____ .

9. Breast development is an early sign of _____ in girls, occurring

between ages 8 and 13; it commonly occurs unilaterally or _____ .

10. During the reproductive years, breasts may become full or tender

in response to hormonal fluctuations during the _____ .

11. During pregnancy, breast changes occur in response to hormones

from the _____ and the _____ .

12. After menopause, breast changes result from a

decrease in _____ levels.

Options
areola
asymmetrically
breast cancer
corpus luteum
estrogen
fatty
fibrous
glandular
lactiferous
lymph
mammary
menstrual cycle
midaxillary
Montgomery's tubercles
nipple
pectoralis major
placenta
puberty
serratus anterior

Here's a gnarly fact: The optimal time to perform a breast self-examination if you're a menstruating woman is 7 to 10 days after menses begins.

A good sports bra...Don't leave home without it!

Finish line

Identify the structures shown in this cross-sectional view of a female breast.

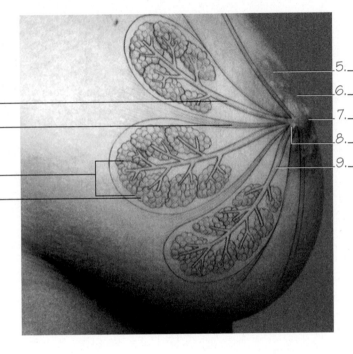

1. _____
2. _____
3. _____
4. _____
5. _____
6. _____
7. _____
8. _____
9. _____

Hit or miss

Indicate whether the following statements about breast structures are true or false.

_____ 1. The tail of Spence is a small triangle of breast tissue that projects into the axilla.

_____ 2. Cooper's ligaments are fibrous tissue bands that attach to the lactiferous ducts.

_____ 3. Milk production occurs in the alveoli within the glandular lobes.

_____ 4. The subscapular lymph nodes drain lymph from most of the anterior chest.

_____ 5. In women, the internal mammary nodes drain lymph from the skin and the superficial lymphatic vessels drain lymph from the mammary lobes.

_____ 6. The nipple and areola are normally pink in all men and women because they contain very little pigment.

■ Finish line

Identify the lymph node chains shown in this illustration.

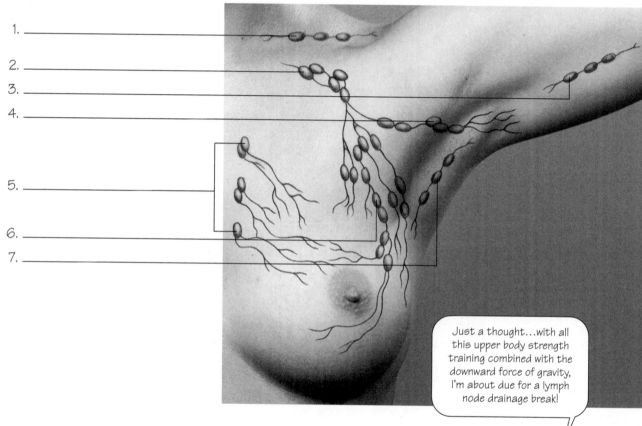

1. _____

2. _____

3. _____

4. _____

5. _____

6. _____

7. _____

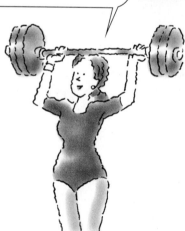

Just a thought...with all this upper body strength training combined with the downward force of gravity, I'm about due for a lymph node drainage break!

■ Brain crunches

Think fast...this one should be easy.

Question: Can you name at least three common breast-related complaints reported by patients during a health history?

1. _____

2. _____

3. _____

■■ ■ Strikeout

Cross out the inappropriate term or phrase in these statements about breast and axillae assessment.

1. Breast skin should be smooth, undimpled, very warm, and the same color as the rest of the skin.

2. Breasts are commonly examined with the patient lying supine with her hand behind her head on the side you're examining, sitting with arms at her sides, holding her arms over her head, lying on her stomach with arms extended to the side, and standing with her hands on the back of a chair while leaning forward.

3. Nipples should be examined for size and shape, discharge, elasticity, reflexes, and protrusion.

4. Nodularity, irregular shape, fullness, and mild tenderness of breasts are common premenstrual symptoms that may be noted during a breast exam.

5. Palpation typically includes gently rotating three fingers in concentric circles against the chest wall, moving from the chest periphery toward the nipple, including the tail of Spence, and gently squeezing the areola and nipple with a gloved hand.

6. Palpable lymph nodes typically are hard, small, and nontender.

■■ ■ You make the call

List the patient's approximate age or developmental stage based on the breast changes illustrated below.

1. _____

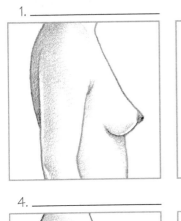

2. _____

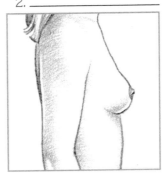

3. _____

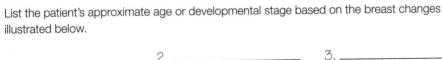
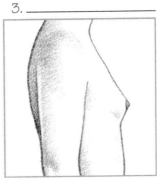

4. _____

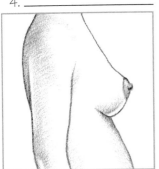

5. _____

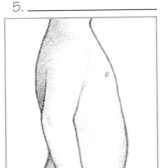

6. _____

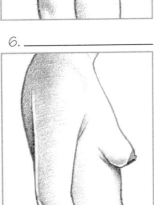

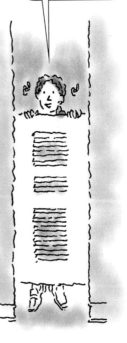

Pardon me while I change...I feel a new developmental stage coming on.

■ Team colors

Using the diagram below, show where you would expect to find a lesion in these areas:

1. Lower inner quadrant at about 7 o'clock
2. Upper outer quadrant at the tail of Spence

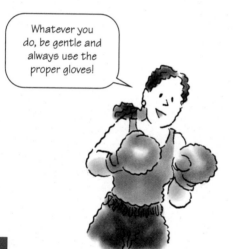

Whatever you do, be gentle and always use the proper gloves!

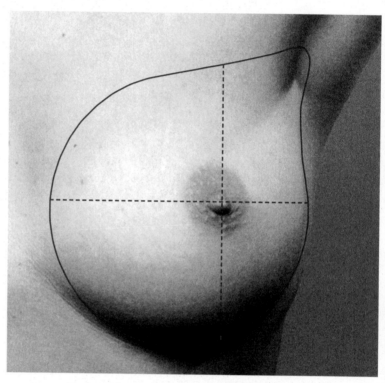

■ Brain crunches

Quick now…the answer to this one should be right at your fingertips.

Question: **If you palpate a mass on your patient's breast, which six characteristics should you record?**

1. _____
2. _____
3. _____
4. _____
5. _____
6. _____

You make the call

Identify the common breast abnormalities pictured here.

1. _____

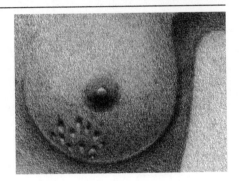

2. _____

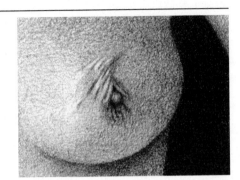

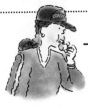

Coaching session

Breasts: A delicate subject

Thanks to more widespread attention in recent years, breast cancer awareness is on the rise and women of all ages are becoming better educated about risk factors, diagnostic measures, and available treatments. But no matter how well informed your patient is, she can still feel anxious during a breast examination. That's because the social and psychological significance of female breasts goes far beyond their biological function. The breast is more than a delicate structure; it's a delicate subject.

During your assessment, it's important to help the patient feel at ease to reduce her anxiety. Provide privacy, make her as comfortable as possible, and explain what the examination involves.

Males have breasts, too

Keep in mind that men also need breast exams, and the incidence of breast cancer in males is rising. Men with breast disorders may feel uneasy or embarrassed about being examined because they see their condition as being unmanly. Remember that a man needs a gentle hand as much as a woman does.

Be sure to examine a man's breasts thoroughly during a complete physical examination. Don't overlook palpation of the nipple and areola; assess for the same changes as you would in a woman. Breast cancer in men usually occurs in the areolar area. Other common breast conditions in males include gynecomastia (more common in older men) and the temporary stimulation of breast tissue caused by estrogen in adolescent boys.

Team up!

Can you differentiate a benign breast lesion from a malignant lesion based on how it feels?
Write these palpation findings under their correct heading and show your stuff!

Benign lesion

_____

_____

_____

_____

_____

Malignant lesion

_____

_____

_____

_____

_____

Palpation findings
- Usually nontender with skin retraction
- Very mobile; feels slippery
- Round and lobular
- Poorly defined edges; feels firm to hard
- Nontender; no skin retraction
- Well-demarcated; feels firm to soft
- Irregular or star-shaped
- Fixed and single

■ Match point

Match the breast finding or disorder in column 1 with its definition or characteristics in column 2.

Breast finding or disorder

1. Peau d'orange _____

2. Gynecomastia _____

3. Mastitis _____

4. Nipple retraction _____

5. Fibrocystic breast disease _____

6. Breast cancer _____

7. Adenofibroma _____

8. Breast dimpling _____

Definition or characteristics

A. Single nodule that feels firm, elastic, and round with well-defined margins and "slippery"; usually found around nipple or lateral side of upper outer quadrant.

B. Painful, red, hot, swollen breast that can cause nipple retraction, deviation, cracking, or flattening; often accompanied by flulike symptoms

C. Abnormal breast enlargement in males; may be hormone-related or caused by cirrhosis, leukemia, thyrotoxicosis, or alcohol or illicit drug use

D. Abnormal puckering of skin, especially around nipple; usually suggests inflammatory or malignant mass beneath skin surface

E. Smooth, round slightly elastic nodules that increase in size just before menstruation; often associated with bloating, irritability, and abdominal cramping

F. Edematous thickening and pitting of breast skin that's commonly a late sign of breast cancer; may also occur with breast or axillary node infection associated with Graves' disease

G. Inward displacement of nipple below level of surrounding tissue; may indicate inflammatory breast lesion or cancer

H. Hard, poorly delineated nodule that's fixed to skin or underlying tissue; may be accompanied by nipple retraction, serous or bloody discharge, or other breast changes

> Well, yes and no...
> Yes, they do make chest binders, support vests, and bras for men. And no, that isn't a silly question.

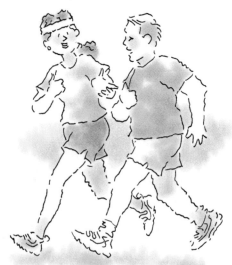

Pep talk

66 Self-confidence is the first requisite to great undertakings. 99
—Samuel Johnson

9

Gastrointestinal system

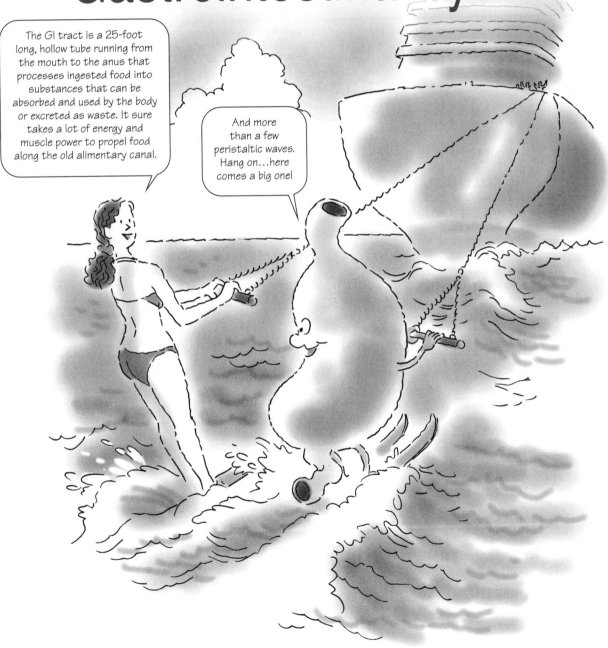

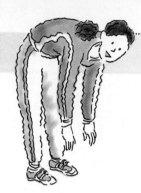

Gastrointestinal system review

Functions

- Ingestion and digestion of food
- Elimination of waste products

Structures

GI tract

- Mouth—responsible for chewing, salivation, and swallowing
- Pharynx—allows passage of food from the mouth to the esophagus
- Epiglottis—closes over larynx when food is swallowed to prevent aspiration into the airway
- Esophagus—moves food from the pharynx to the stomach
- Stomach—serves as a reservoir for food and secretes gastric juices that aid in digestion
- Small intestine—consists of the duodenum, the jejunum, and the ileum; absorbs end products of digestion into the bloodstream and digests carbohydrates, fats, and proteins
- Large intestine—consists of the cecum; the ascending, transverse, descending, and sigmoid colons; the rectum; and the anus; responsible for absorbing excess water and electrolytes, storing food residue, and eliminating waste products

Accessory organs

- Liver—metabolizes carbohydrates, fats, and proteins; detoxifies the blood; converts ammonia to urea; and synthesizes proteins and essential nutrients
- Gallbladder—stores bile from the liver until it's emptied into the duodenum
- Pancreas—releases insulin and glycogen into the bloodstream; secretes pancreatic enzymes that aid digestion
- Bile ducts—serve as passageways for bile from the liver to the intestines
- Abdominal aorta—supplies blood to the GI tract

Health history

Ask the patient about:

- past GI illnesses, surgery, and trauma
- medications, including laxative use
- current GI signs or symptoms
- family medical history, especially history of ulcerative colitis, colorectal cancer, peptic ulcers, and gastric cancer
- diet, exercise patterns, and alcohol, caffeine, and tobacco use.

Assessment

Mouth

- Inspect the mouth and jaw as well as the inner and outer lips, teeth, gums, and oral mucosa.
- Inspect the tongue.
- Palpate for areas of tenderness or lesions.

Abdomen

- Inspect the abdomen for symmetry, shape, and contour.
- Note abdominal movements and pulsations.
- Auscultate in each of the four abdominal quadrants to assess bowel sounds and over the abdominal arteries to check for bruits, venous hums, and friction rubs.
- Percuss the abdomen, listening for tympany over hollow organs (such as an empty stomach or intestine) and for dullness over solid organs (such as the liver) or feces-filled intestines.
- Palpate in all four quadrants of the abdomen, leaving painful areas for last.
- Check for rebound tenderness if you suspect peritoneal inflammation; also check for ascites, a large accumulation of fluid in the peritoneal cavity.

Rectum and anus

- Inspect the perianal area.
- Palpate the rectum using a water-soluble lubricant on your gloved index finger.

Abnormal findings

- Nausea and vomiting—may be caused by existing illness or by certain medications
- Dysphagia—difficulty swallowing; has various causes; may lead to aspiration and pneumonia
- Cullen's sign—a bluish umbilicus; indicates intra-abdominal hemorrhage
- Turner's sign—bruising on the flank; indicates retroperitoneal hemorrhage
- Constipation—may occur with a dull abdominal ache, a full feeling, and hyperactive bowel sounds
- Diarrhea—may occur with cramping, abdominal tenderness, anorexia, and hyperactive bowel sounds
- Abdominal distention—may occur with gas, a tumor, or a colon filled with feces
- Abnormal bowels sounds—may be hyperactive (indicating increased intestinal motility) or hypoactive
- Friction rubs—may indicate splenic infarction or hepatic tumor
- Abdominal pain—may result from ulcers, intestinal obstruction, appendicitis, cholecystitis, peritonitis, or other inflammatory disorders

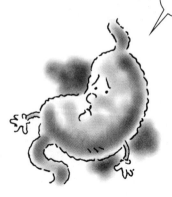

A disruption of the function of the GI system can cause problems ranging from loss of appetite to acid-base imbalances. Stomach pain, nausea, and vomiting strongly suggest a GI problem.

Since you've just finished reviewing key concepts about the GI system, this exercise shouldn't be too much of a mind stretch.

■ Batter's box

Here's an easy anatomy and physiology exercise to get you started on the GI tract. Simply fill in the blanks with the appropriate words.

Trekking down the GI tract

The GI tract begins at the _____ and ends at the _____ and
                                        1   2

consists of smooth muscle, blood vessels, and nerve tissue. Food is propelled along the tract

by _____ . GI organs include the pharynx, or throat, the _____ , a
              3

hollow, muscular tube which moves food from the pharynx to the stomach, the stomach, and
        4

the small and large _____ .
                                                    5

　　The stomach has three main functions: storing food, mixing food with gastric juices, and

passing _____ , a watery mixture of partly digested food and digestive juices.
                    6

The small intestine breaks down food into _____ , fats, and proteins. The large
                                                                        7

intestine, or _____ , absorbs excess water and electrolytes, stores food residue,
                          8

and eliminates wastes in the form of _____ .
                                                              9

Don't forget your accessories

The _____ , the body's heaviest organ, metabolizes carbohydrates, fats, and
              10

proteins; detoxifies blood; and synthesizies various substances. It also secretes

_____ , a greenish fluid that helps digest fats.
        11

　　Other major accessory organs include the _____ , which stores bile secret-
                                                                      12

ed by the liver, and the _____ , which releases insulin and glycogen into the
                                        13

bloodstream.

Options

anus

bile

carbohydrates

chyme

colon

esophagus

feces

gallbladder

intestines

liver

mouth

pancreas

peristalsis

Jumble gym

Unscramble the words below to discover signs and symptoms commonly reported during the health history interview. Then use the circled letters to answer the question.

Question: The loud, gurgling, splashing bowel sound heard when gas passes through the large intestine is called what? (*Hint:* You might know it by its common name—a growling stomach.)

1. B E A T H R U N R   _ _ _ _ _ ◯ _ _ _

2. L A R T E C   G I D B E N E L   ◯ _ _ _ _ _   ◯ _ _ _ _ _ _

3. E N A S A U   _ _ _ ◯ _ _

4. C L A U N F L E E T   _ _ _ _ _ ◯ _ _ _ _

5. V I M I O T N G   _ ◯ _ _ _ _ _ ◯

6. H E A D A R I R   _ _ _ _ ◯ _ _ _

7. G A I H Y P A D S   _ ◯ _ _ _ _ _ _

8. T O N S T O P C A I N I   _ ◯ _ _ _ _ _ _ _ _ _

9. H A S T E C A M H O C   _ _ _ ◯ _ _ _ _ _

Answer: _ _ _ _ _ _ _ _ _ _ _ _

I went the distance, but I can't stop here...gotta find a bathroom quick!

Mind sprints

If your patient is complaining of diarrhea, go the distance to learn as much as you can during the health history interview. Time yourself, and see how many questions you can list in 5 minutes.

_____
_____
_____
_____
_____
_____
_____
_____
_____
_____
_____
_____

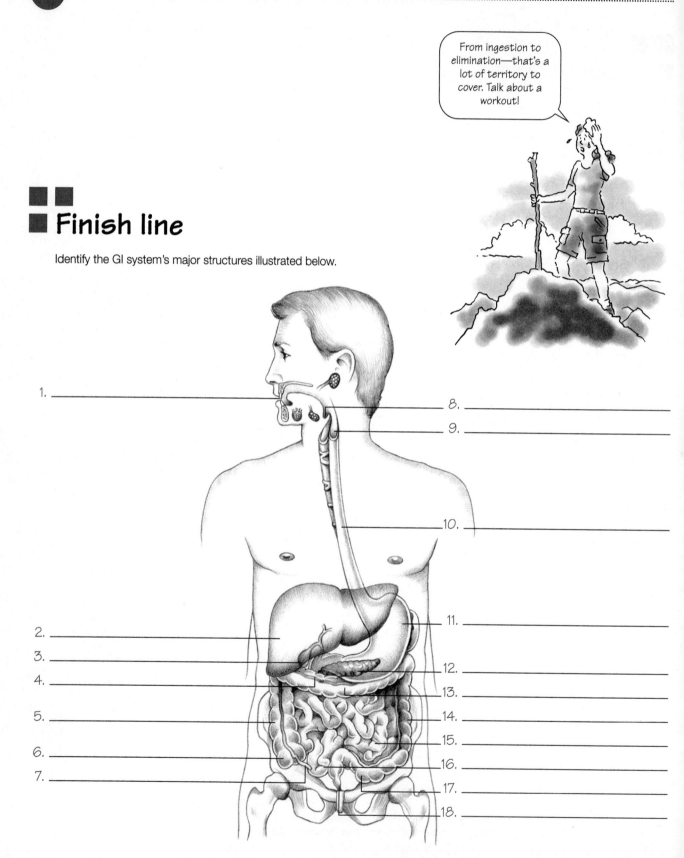

■■
■ Finish line

Identify the GI system's major structures illustrated below.

From ingestion to elimination—that's a lot of territory to cover. Talk about a workout!

1. _____

2. _____

3. _____

4. _____

5. _____

6. _____

7. _____

8. _____

9. _____

10. _____

11. _____

12. _____

13. _____

14. _____

15. _____

16. _____

17. _____

18. _____

■■ Brain crunches

Hustle now, and work those brain cells to answer this question.

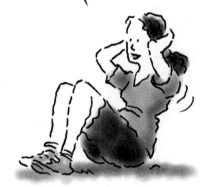

No, I'm not working on my six-pack abs...just hoping to move my breakfast along.

Question: **Can you name at least five GI disorders that have a familial link?**

1. _____
2. _____
3. _____
4. _____
5. _____

■■ Strikeout

Get the skinny on your patient's GI health by focusing on the right information during the health history interview. Cross out the term or phrase that doesn't belong in each of the following questions.

1. Have you ever been diagnosed with a GI illness, such as an ulcer, inflammatory bowel disease, von Willebrand's disease, irritable bowel syndrome, or gastroesophageal reflux?

2. Are you currently taking any multivitamins, aspirin, nonsteroidal anti-inflammatory drugs, antibiotics, or opioid analgesics?

3. Have you noticed any changes in appetite, ability to chew or swallow, bowel habits, or resistance to disease?

4. What's your usual diet, exercise routine, sexual pattern, sleep pattern, and oral hygiene?

5. Do you have any allergies to pets, foods, or medicines?

6. Have you noticed any changes in the color, odor, temperature, amount, or appearance of your stool?

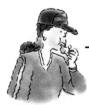

Coaching session
Culture counts, too

When taking a health history, consider your patient's ethnic background. For example, patients from Japan, Iceland, Chile, and Austria are at higher risk of death from gastric cancer than patients from other countries. Also, Crohn's disease is more common in patients who are Jewish.

Batter's box

You'll need to stretch your memory of GI assessment techniques for this game. Fill in the blanks with the correct words to complete the 10 techique tips provided here.

> Ten-minute penalty for roughing the abdomen (palpating before auscultating)!

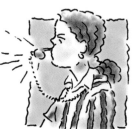

1. During a physical examination of the GI system, thoroughly inspect the

_____ , _____ , and _____ .

2. Follow this sequence to perform an abdominal assessment: inspection,

_____ , _____ , and _____ .

3. Use the techniques of _____ and palpation to assess the

mouth.

4. Begin your inspection of the abdomen by first mentally dividing it into four

_____ .

5. When assessing the *epigastric* area, focus on the structures above the

_____ and between the _____ .

6. When assessing the *umbilical* region, concentrate around the

_____ ; when checking the *suprapubic* area, focus above the

_____ .

7. Classify bowel sounds as _____ , _____ , or

_____ .

8. Anticipate normal bowel sounds to be loudest _____ .

9. Remember that percussion is used to detect the size and location of abdomi-

nal organs and to detect _____ or _____ in the ab-

domen, stomach, or bowel.

10. Always palpate the abdomen in a _____ direction.

Options
abdomen
air
auscultation
before mealtimes
clockwise
costal margins
fluid
hyperactive
hypoactive
inspection
mouth
navel
normal
palpation
percussion
quadrants
rectum
symphysis pubis
umbilicus

■ Match point

When assessing the GI system, begin at the source by examining the oral cavity.
Match the oral structure in column 1 with what you're assessing for in column 2.

Oral structure

1. Gums, inner lips, and cheeks _____
2. Tongue _____
3. Mouth and jaw _____
4. Pharynx _____

Assessing for

A. Coating, tremors, swelling, and ulcerations
B. Asymmetry, swelling, and malocclusion
C. Uvular deviation, tonsillar abnormalities, lesions, plaques, and exudate
D. Tenderness, lumps, and lesions

■ You make the call

List the abdominal structures found in each quadrant under their corresponding headings.

Right upper quadrant

_____
_____
_____
_____
_____
_____

Left upper quadrant

_____
_____
_____
_____

Right lower quadrant

_____
_____

Left lower quadrant

_____
_____

Sometimes you have to divide and conquer to get the job done.

Gear up!

Did you bring all the right equipment for the exam? Check off which equipment or supplies you'll need to perform a routine physical examination of the GI system.

☐ Stethoscope
☐ Gloves
☐ Cotton-tipped applicators
☐ Lubricant
☐ Otoscope
☐ Ruler (in centimeters)
☐ Flexible tape measure
☐ Blood pressure cuff
☐ Snellen chart
☐ Urine specimen container
☐ Guaiac test kit
☐ Forceps
☐ Syringe

☐ Pen
☐ Scale
☐ Tongue blade
☐ Thermometer
☐ Mirror
☐ Tuning fork
☐ Safety pin
☐ Penlight
☐ Speculum
☐ Drape
☐ Small pillow
☐ Percussion hammer

Unless I'm undergoing a laparoscopy, I don't think we'll need this!

Match point

Match the normal finding in column 1 with the abdominal assessment in column 2.

Normal finding

1. Smooth, uniform color _____
2. Flat to rounded, or slightly concave _____
3. Inverted and midline _____
4. None or only slight _____
5. High-pitched and gurgling _____
6. Tympanic or dull _____

Abdominal assessment

A. Abdominal pulsations
B. Bowel sounds
C. Abdominal skin
D. Abdominal percussion
E. Abdominal shape
F. Umbilicus

Team up!

Are your patient's bowel sounds hyperactive or hypoactive, and do you know what causes them? Show us you have what it takes by teaming up the cause under the appropriate heading.

Hyperactive bowel sounds

_____

_____

_____

_____

_____

Hypoactive bowel sounds

_____

_____

_____

_____

_____

Common causes
- Use of opioid analgesics
- Diarrhea
- Laxative use
- Peritonitis
- Ileus
- Constipation
- Bowel obstruction or torsion

No worries! That tinkling sound you hear is me giving the old ivories a workout— not hyperactive bowel sounds.

You make the call

Vascular sounds may be auscultated over all of the abdominal areas indicated in this illustration. Name the arterial sites.

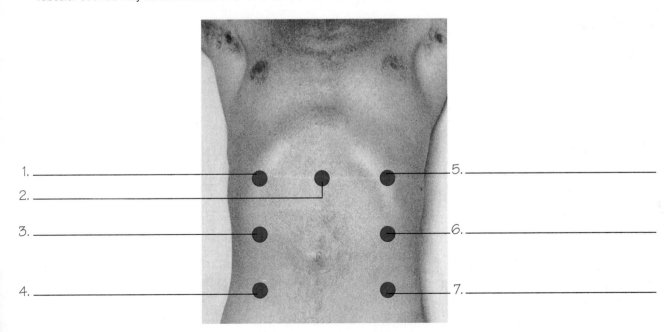

1. _____

2. _____

3. _____

4. _____

5. _____

6. _____

7. _____

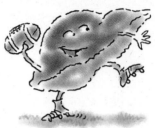

I'm sure you'll know the answer to this one. Just reach back, and let 'er rip!

■■ You make the call

Is it tympany or dullness you hear when percussing your patient's abdomen? Identify which sound you're likely to hear over each of the areas shown in the illustration, and explain why the sound occurs.

1. Small circled area: _____
_____
_____
_____
_____

2. Large circled area: _____
_____
_____
_____
_____

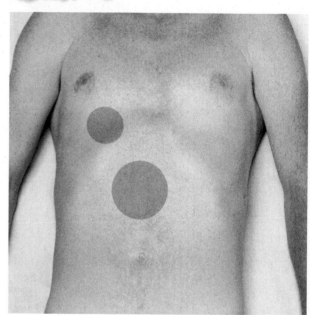

■■ Step aerobics

Identify what abdominal assessment the nurse is performing in this photo, and briefly describe the steps involved.

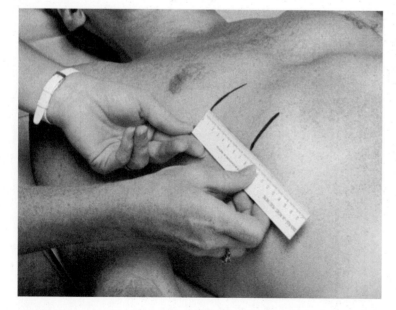

Assessment: _____
_____

Procedure steps:

1. _____
_____
_____

2. _____
_____
_____

3. _____
_____
_____

> **Pep talk**
>
> Let proportion be found not only in numbers and measures, but also in sounds, weights, times, and positions, and whatever force there is.
>
> —Leonardo da Vinci

■ Hit or miss

Indicate whether the following statements are true or false.

_____ 1. Splenomegaly may be caused by mononucleosis, trauma, or illnesses that destroy red blood cells, such as sickle cell anemia.

_____ 2. Before auscultating the abdomen of a patient with a nasogastric tube or another abdominal tube connected to suction, briefly clamp the tube or turn off suction because noises can obscure or mimic bowel sounds.

_____ 3. Auscultate with the diaphragm of the stethoscope over the aorta and renal, iliac, and femoral arteries to hear bruits, venous hums, and friction rubs.

_____ 4. Percussing the abdomen of a patient with an abdominal aneurysm or a transplanted abdominal organ can precipitate a rupture or organ rejection.

_____ 5. You should always palpate painful or tender abdominal organs first.

_____ 6. Deep palpation helps identify muscle resistance and tenderness as well as the location of superficial organs.

_____ 7. Unless the patient's spleen is large, it isn't palpable.

_____ 8. To perform light palpation, depress the abdomen about ½″ (1.5 cm); to perform deep palpation, depress about 4″ to 5″ (10 to 13 cm)

_____ 9. It's okay to palpate a rigid abdomen as long as the patient isn't in pain.

_____ 10. Palpation is used to help estimate the size of a patient's liver.

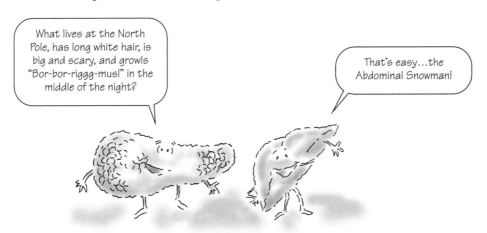

What lives at the North Pole, has long white hair, is big and scary, and growls "Bor-bor-rigg-mus!" in the middle of the night?

That's easy...the Abdominal Snowman!

Cross-training

Work these clues to test your knowledge of the GI system and assessment findings.

Across

1. Large intestine
2. Marked lines that sometimes appear on abdomen from pregnancy, weight gain, or ascites
4. Large amount of fluid in abdominal cavity
9. Thin, leaf-shaped structure that helps prevent aspiration of swallowed food or air
11. Usually can't be palpated unless it's enlarged
12. Habitual use of these can cause constipation

Down

1. Part of large intestine found in right lower quadrant
2. Liquid produced by parotid, submandibular, and sublingual glands
3. Muscular, hollow tube between pharynx and stomach
5. Wavelike movement of food through intestines
6. Infrequently heard bowel sounds
7. Around the navel
8. Saclike reservoir found in the left upper quadrant
10. Organ that lies horizontally in abdomen, behind the stomach

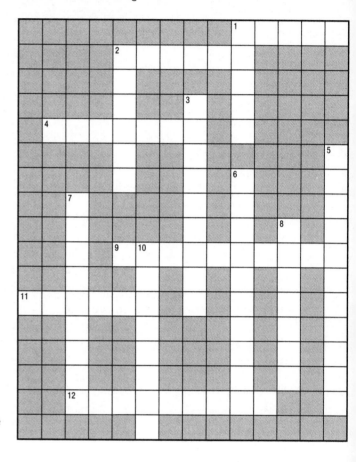

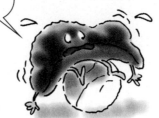

Are you sure this is the best workout for a tender organ like me?

You make the call

Identify the examination techniques shown in these illustrations, and tell which organ they're used to assess.

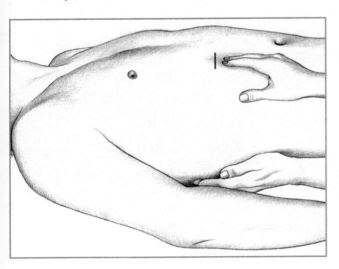

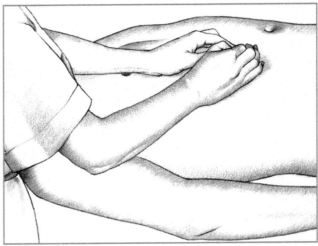

1. _____

_____

_____

_____

2. _____

_____

_____

_____

Match point

Match the GI assessment term in column 1 with its definition in column 2.

GI assessment term

1. Hepatomegaly _____

2. Positive splenic percussion sign _____

3. Splenomegaly _____

4. Ascites _____

5. Rebound tenderness _____

6. Paralytic ileus _____

Definition

A. Enlargement of the spleen

B. Absent or limited passage due to paralysis of the bowel

C. Change from tympany to dullness that's noted upon assessment of the area between the 9th and 11th intercostal spaces when patient breathes deeply

D. Enlargement of the liver

E. Excess fluid in the abdominal cavity

F. Painful response that's elicited upon removal of pressure applied to the abdomen

You make the call

Identify the assessment technique shown in this picture, and briefly explain how it's done.

Assessment technique: _____

_____

How it's done: _____

_____

_____

_____

_____

_____

_____

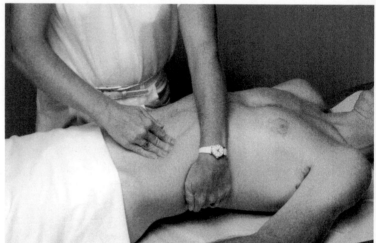

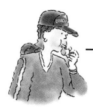

Coaching session
Eliciting rebound tenderness in children

Eliciting rebound tenderness in young children who can't verbalize how they feel may be difficult. Be alert for such clues as an anguished facial expression, grimace, or intensified crying.

When attempting to assess this symptom, use techniques that elicit minimal tenderness. For example, have the child hop or jump to allow tissue to rebound gently while you watch for signs of pain. With this technique, the child won't associate the exacerbation of his pain with your actions, and you may gain the child's cooperation.

Train your brain

Sound out each group of pictures to reveal terms that complete this assessment consideration.

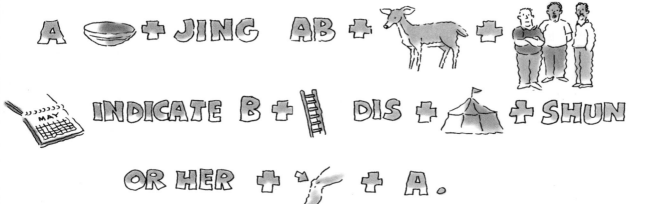

Answer: _____

You make the call

Now here's an unusual-looking assessment procedure. Identify what it is and how it's performed.

Assessment technique: _____

_____

How it's done: _____

_____

_____

_____

_____

_____

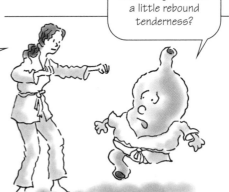

■ Choose the best course

Fill in the boxes to show the correct sequence used when performing a rectal examination.

Steps

After applying water-soluble lubricant to index finger, insert finger, aiming toward umbilicus.

Ask patient to strain as if having a bowel movement.

Inspect the perianal area.

Inspect glove for stool, blood, and mucus and test fecal matter with a guaiac test.

Put on gloves.

Spread buttocks to expose anus and surrounding tissue, and check for abnormalities.

Palpate rectum in a clockwise, then a counterclockwise direction.

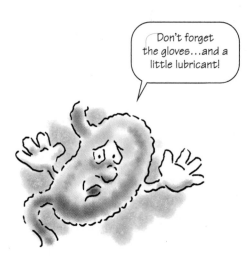

Don't forget the gloves...and a little lubricant!

Brain crunches

Here we go again! Answer this one as fast as you can.

Question: Can you name 10 abnormalities you might find during a rectal examination—hopefully, not all at the same time?

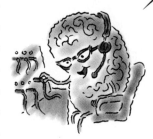

The buzz is you're doing wonderfully with all these exercises. Keep up the good work!

1. _____
2. _____
3. _____
4. _____
5. _____
6. _____
7. _____
8. _____
9. _____
10. _____

Match point

Words used to describe abdominal pain can provide clues about the probable cause.
Match the descriptive word in column 1 with the likely cause of pain in column 2.

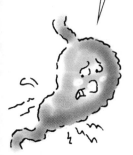

Does "OWWWW!" qualify as a good descriptive word?

Descriptive word

1. Burning _____
2. Cramping _____
3. Severe cramping _____
4. Stabbing _____

Likely cause of pain

A. Appendicitis, Crohn's disease, diverticulitis

B. Biliary colic, irritable bowel syndrome, diarrhea, flatulence

C. Peptic ulcer, gastroesophageal reflux

D. Pancreatitis, cholecystitis

■ Batter's box

Aerobicize your brain cells by filling in the appropriate words in this review of GI signs and symptoms.

1. Dysphagia can lead to aspiration and _____ .

2. Diarrhea that occurs within several hours of ingesting milk or milk products may be a sign of _____ .

3. Flank bruising, or _____ sign, is an indication of retroperitoneal hemorrhage.

4. A _____ ulcer can cause gnawing abdominal pain in the epigastrium 1½ to 3 hours after eating.

5. The passage of bloody stools is known as _____ .

6. _____ tends to occur more commonly in elderly patients and in those who are immobile or sedentary.

7. A bluish umbilicus, or _____ sign, indicates intra-abdominal hemorrhage.

8. Protrusion of the umbilicus when the patient raises his head and shoulders may be caused by an _____ .

9. Visible rippling peristaltic waves over the abdomen may indicate _____ and should be reported immediately.

10. Perform a test for rebound tenderness whenever you suspect _____ inflammation.

11. Hepatomegaly and cutaneous angiomas may signal _____ disease.

Options

bowel obstruction

constipation

Cullen's

duodenal

hematochezia

lactose intolerance

liver

peritoneal

pneumonia

Turner's

umbilical hernia

Strikeout

Cross out the term or phrase that doesn't belong in these statements about assessment findings and GI conditions.

1. During palpation of the rectum, the rectal walls should normally feel soft and smooth, mucous or bloody, and without masses or fecal impaction.

2. Dysphagia can be caused by an obstruction, achalasia of the lower esophagogastric junction, stroke, Parkinson's disease, or dysmenorrhea.

3. Ascites can be caused by thyrotoxicosis, advanced liver disease, heart failure, pancreatitis, or cancer.

4. Hyperactive bowel sounds unrelated to hunger may be caused by diarrhea, laxative use, early bowel obstruction, or paralytic ileus.

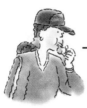

Coaching session

Differentiating spleen and kidney enlargement

To differentiate between spleen and kidney enlargement, ask your patient to take a deep breath. Then percuss along the 9th and 11th intercostal spaces. You should hear tympany produced by colonic or gastric air. If you hear dullness instead, the patient's spleen may be enlarged. If you hear resonance, his left kidney may be enlarged.

If you hear resonance instead of tympany when percussing along the 9th and 11th intercostal spaces, you're probably sensing a bulkier me. Wish I could say that my enlargement is due to weight training, but it's probably a sign of a problem that needs further investigation.

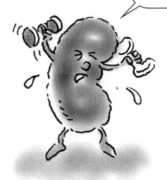

Match point

Match the findings in column 1 with the corresponding disorder or probable cause in column 2.

Findings

1. Right lower quadrant pain accompanied by increased abdominal wall resistance and guarding _____

2. Dilated, tortuous, visible abdominal veins _____

3. Nausea and vomiting of undigested food, diarrhea, abdominal cramping, hyperactive bowel sounds, and fever _____

4. Bright-red rectal bleeding, diarrhea or ribbon-shaped (possibly bloody) stools, weakness and fatigue, abdominal aching and cramps _____

5. Chronic, sometimes painful bleeding with defecation _____

6. Soft, unformed stools or watery (possibly foul-smelling) diarrhea; abdominal pain, cramping, and tenderness; and fever _____

7. Recurrent bloody diarrhea with pus or mucus, hyperactive bowel sounds, and occasional nausea and vomiting _____

8. Diarrhea that occurs within hours after consuming milk or milk products; abdominal pain, cramping, and bloating; borborygmus; and flatulence _____

9. Moderate to severe rectal bleeding, epistaxis, and purpura _____

Corresponding disorder or probable cause

A. Hemorrhoids

B. Lactose intolerance

C. Gastroenteritis

D. Ulcerative colitis

E. Appendicitis

F. Colon cancer

G. Inferior vena cava obstruction

H. Coagulation disorders

I. *Clostridium difficile* infection

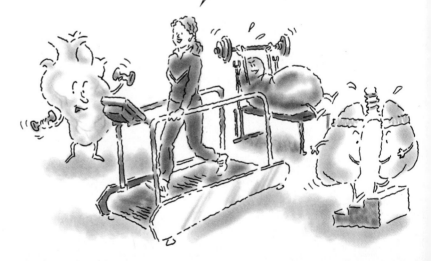

I'm so impressed with how you're keeping up! Get ready to move on to the next workout station...er, chapter...it's coming up fast.

Female genitourinary system

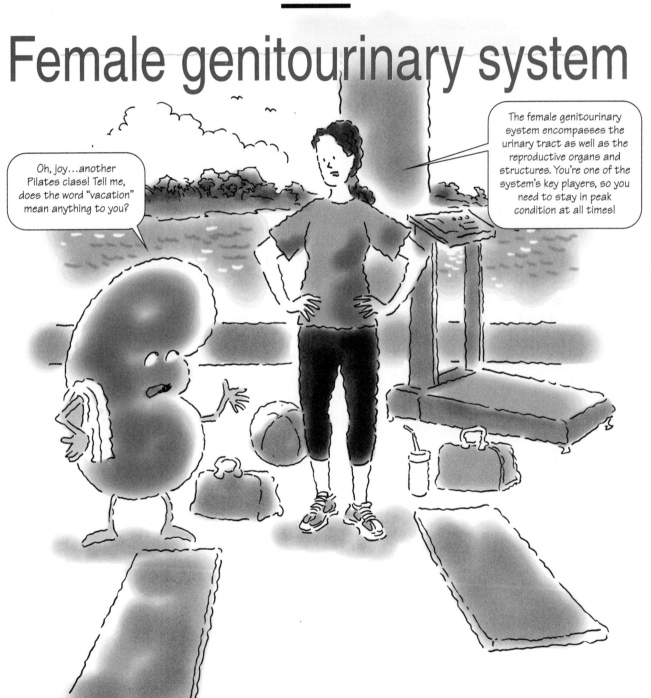

Female genitourinary system review

Structures of the urinary system

■ Kidneys—form urine; maintain homeostasis; contain nephrons
■ Ureters—carry urine from the kidneys to the bladder
■ Bladder—container for urine collection
■ Urethra—carries urine from the bladder to outside of the body

Structures of the internal genitalia

■ Vagina—route of passage for childbirth and menstruation
■ Uterus—nurtures and then expels the fetus during pregnancy; divided into the fundus and cervix
■ Ovaries—produce ova and release the hormones estrogen and progesterone
■ Fallopian tubes—the usual site of fertilization of the ova by the sperm; help to guide the ova to the uterus after expulsion from the ovaries

Health history

Ask about:
■ urinary tract infections, kidney disease or kidney stones, and past medical history
■ menstruation and sexual practices
■ pregnancy and birth control
■ menopause.

Assessment

Urinary system

■ Inspect the areas over the kidneys and bladder.
■ Percuss the kidneys (to check for costovertebral angle tenderness) and bladder.
■ Attempt to palpate the kidneys and bladder. (They aren't normally palpable unless the kidneys are enlarged or the bladder is distended.)

Reproductive system

■ Inspect the external genitalia; note the appearance of pubic hair to determine sexual maturity.
■ Palpate the external genitalia—this should be pain-free for the patient.
■ Inspect internal genitalia using a speculum lubricated with warm water.
■ Examine the vaginal wall for color, texture, and integrity and the cervix for color, position, size, shape, mucosal integrity, and discharge.
■ Palpate the internal genitalia, including bimanual palpation and rectovaginal palpation.

> Remember that the kidneys and bladder aren't normally palpable unless the kidneys are enlarged or the bladder is distended.

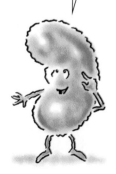

Abnormal findings

Urinary system

- Polyuria—overproduction of urine
- Hematuria—blood in the urine, causing urine to turn brown or bright red
- Urinary frequency—abnormally frequent urination
- Urinary urgency—sudden urge to urinate
- Urinary hesitancy—difficulty starting urine stream
- Nocturia—excessive urination at night
- Urinary incontinence—involuntary release of urine
- Dysuria—painful urination

Reproductive system

- Genital lesions—may result from syphilis (red, painless, eroding lesion with a raised, indurated border), genital warts (painless, tiny, red or pink swellings that develop stemlike structures), or genital herpes (multiple, shallow vesicles, lesions, or crusts)
- Vaginal discharge—may result from bacterial vaginosis (thin, grayish white discharge), *Candida albicans* (thick, white, curdlike discharge), trichomoniasis (malodorous, yellow or green, and watery or frothy discharge), chlamydia (mucopurulent discharge), or gonorrhea (purulent green-yellow discharge)

- Cervical polyps—bright, red, soft, and fragile lesions
- Vaginal and uterine prolapse—anterior vaginal wall and bladder prolapse into the vagina
- Rectocele—herniation of the rectum through the posterior vaginal wall
- Dysmenorrhea—painful menstruation
- Amenorrhea—absence of menstrual flow

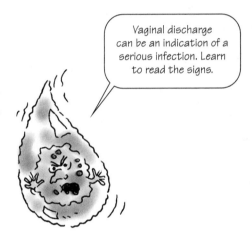

Vaginal discharge can be an indication of a serious infection. Learn to read the signs.

■ Hit or miss

Indicate whether the following statements about the female genitourinary system are true or false.

_____ 1. The female genitourinary system encompasses the urinary tract and the reproductive organs and structures. Major structures of the urinary system include the kidneys, ureters, bladder, vagina, and urethra.

_____ 2. The primary functions of the urinary system include forming urine and maintaining the proper balance of fluids, minerals, and organic substances for homeostasis.

_____ 3. The kidneys are located retroperitoneally on either side of the thoracic vertebrae, behind the abdominal organs.

_____ 4. Urine gathers in the collecting tubules and ducts of the nephrons and drains into the ureters, down into the bladder, and out through the urethra.

_____ 5. The external genitalia, or vulva, include the mons pubis, labia majora and minora, clitoris, vagina, urethra, and Skene's and Bartholin's glands.

_____ 6. The vagina is a hollow, collapsed tube that extends from the vulva to the uterus.

_____ 7. The uterus, a hollow, pear-shaped organ, is divided into the cervix (upper portion of the uterus) and the fundus, which protrudes into the vagina; its primary purpose is to nurture and expel the fetus during pregnancy.

_____ 8. The ovaries produce ova (eggs) and release the hormones estrogen and epinephrine.

_____ 9. The fallopian tubes extend from the ovaries to the upper portion of the uterus and help guide the ova after expulsion by the ovaries.

_____ 10. Fertilization of the ova by sperm usually occurs in the uterine cavity.

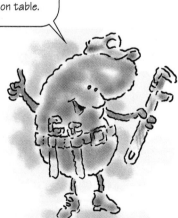

The good news is no leaks and everything seems to be in good working order. The bad news is my bill…I left it by the examination table.

Finish line

Identify the main structures of the urinary system shown in this illustration.

1. _____

2. _____

3. _____

4. _____

5. _____

6. _____

7. _____

8. _____

In the ballpark

Let's see how well you know your female genitourinary statistics. Match the normal range or finding in column 1 with its corresponding structure in column 2.

Normal range or finding

1. 4½″ to 5″ (11.5 to 12.5 cm) long and 2½″ (6.4 cm) wide _____

2. 500 to 1,000 ml _____

3. 1″ to 2″ (2.5 to 5 cm) long _____

4. 4″ (10 cm) long _____

5. 6 to 31 _____

6. 10″ to 12″ (25.5 to 30.5 cm) long and ⅛″ to ¼″ (3 to 6 mm) in diameter _____

7. 1,000,000 _____

Corresponding structure

A. Bladder capacity

B. Ducts in Skene's gland

C. Ureter

D. Nephrons in kidney

E. Urethra

F. Kidney

G. Fallopian tube

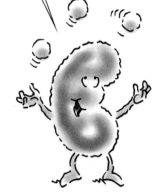

Better to have a slew of ballpark estimates in your game plan than an arsenal of wild pitches, I always say!

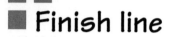

Finish line

Now identify the main parts of the external and internal female genitalia shown in the illustrations below.

External genitalia

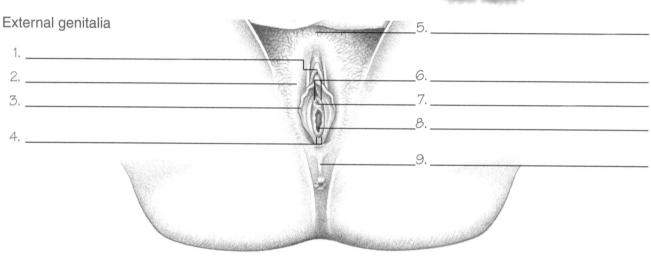

1. _____
2. _____
3. _____
4. _____

5. _____
6. _____
7. _____
8. _____
9. _____

Internal genitalia

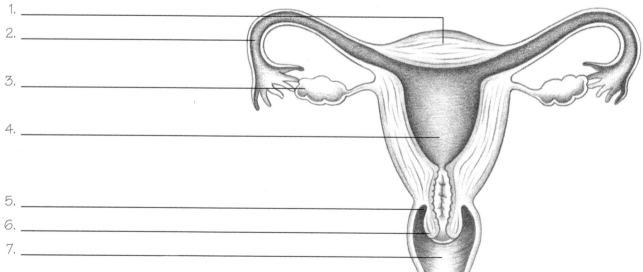

1. _____
2. _____
3. _____
4. _____
5. _____
6. _____
7. _____

Brain crunches

Channel your brainwave energy, and answer this question as quickly as you can.

Question: What are the four most common complaints concerning the urinary system reported by patients?

1. _____

2. _____

3. _____

4. _____

> **Pep talk**
>
> " Don't be too timid and squeamish about your actions. All life is an experiment. The more experiments you make, the better. "
> —Ralph Waldo Emerson

Jumble gym

Unscramble each word to discover terms related to the patient's urinary history.
Then use the circled letters to answer the question below.

Question: A history that includes any of the following past illnesses or preexisting conditions can adversely affect your patient's what?

1. D I N K E Y   O N S E T S   _ _ _ _ _ Ⓞ _ Ⓞ_ Ⓞ_ _

2. P R E T O Y H N I N E S   Ⓞ _ _ _ ⓄⓄ _ _ _ _ _ _ _

3. B E S T A I D E   _ _ _ _ _ Ⓞ _ _

4. A C E G R I L L   A C E I N T R O S
Ⓞ_Ⓞ_ _ _Ⓞ_   Ⓞ_ _ _ _ _ _ _ _

5. R A I N U Y R   A T T R C   F I T S O N I C E
Ⓞ_ _ _ _ _ _   _ _Ⓞ_ _   _ _ _ _Ⓞ_ _ _ _ _

6. A C C R U A L A D V I S O R   S E A S I D E
_ _Ⓞ_ _ _ _Ⓞ_ _ _ _ _   _ _ _ _ _ _ _

7. C H I N O E X P O R T   S U D G R
_Ⓞ_Ⓞ_ _ _ _ _ _   _ _ _ _ _

Answer: _ _ _ _ _ _ _ _   _ _ _ _ _ _   _ _ _ _ _

Brain crunches

Here we go again. We need five more answers…quick as you can.

Question: **List the five most commonly reported reproductive system complaints.**

1. _____

2. _____

3. _____

4. _____

5. _____

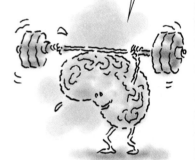

Thomas Edison once said, "Genius is one percent inspiration and ninety-nine percent perspiration." I'm waiting for the 1% to kick in!

Mind sprints

List some questions below that you should ask your patient if you want to learn more about her reproductive system history and potential problems. You have 3 minutes. Ready, set, go!

_____

_____

_____

_____

_____

_____

_____

_____

_____

_____

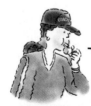

Coaching session
How ethnicity affects menstruation

Studies have shown that a patient's ethnicity has a strong influence on the duration and heaviness of bleeding during menses. Black females tend to have longer menses than white females of the same age. They're also more likely to have a heavier menstrual flow than white females. However, keep in mind that a patient's diet, exercise habits, and stress level may also influence the duration and heaviness of menstruation.

Gear up!

Don't worry…nothing to break a sweat over yet. Simply check off which equipment and supplies you'll need to perform a genitourinary assessment.

- ☐ Gloves
- ☐ Penlight
- ☐ Percussion hammer
- ☐ Blood pressure cuff
- ☐ Vaginal speculum
- ☐ Water-soluble lubricant
- ☐ Specimen containers
- ☐ Cotton-tipped applicators
- ☐ Tongue blade
- ☐ Tuning fork
- ☐ Scale

- ☐ Body mass index chart
- ☐ Otoscope
- ☐ Guaiac test kit
- ☐ Ophthalmoscope
- ☐ Dextrostix kit
- ☐ Gown and drape
- ☐ 20-gauge needle
- ☐ Syringes
- ☐ Tape measure
- ☐ Povidone-iodine solution
- ☐ Warm water

> **Pep talk**
>
> " To invent, you need a good imagination and a pile of junk.
> —Thomas Alva Edison "

Train your brain

Sound out each group of pictures to reveal terms that complete this assessment consideration.

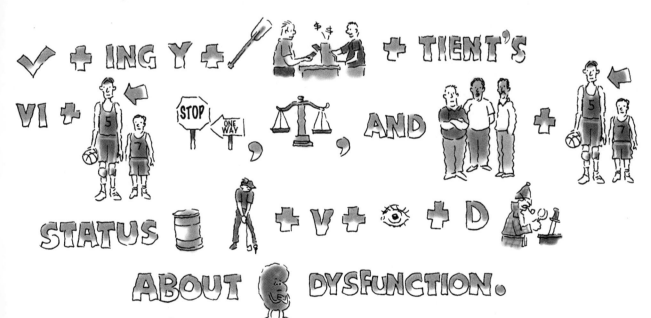

Answer: _____

Strikeout

Cross out the term or phrase that doesn't belong in these statements about performing a female genitourinary assessment.

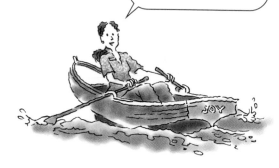

This exercise shouldn't be too much of a strain. Just a few easy pen strokes, and you'll be drifting on to the next activity in no time!

1. Normally, the skin over the kidney and bladder areas should be free from lesions, hair follicles, discoloration, inflammation, and swelling.

2. Normal external genital discharge may be clear and stretchy, white and opaque, or yellow and curdlike depending on the time of the patient's menstrual cycle.

3. You should notify the practitioner and obtain a specimen if the patient's vestibule (especially around the Skene's and Bartholin's glands) shows any signs of swelling, pinkness, lesions, discharge, or unusual odor.

4. Inspection of the patient's umbilicus, external genitalia, and pubic hair can help to assess her sexual maturity.

5. It's possible to milk and culture discharge from the patient's urethra, clitoris, Skene's glands, and Bartholin's glands when these areas are swollen, inflamed, or tender.

6. Common types of specula used to inspect internal genitalia include Pederson, Graves', plastic, and Nagashima Takahashi varieties.

7. The cervix is commonly examined for color, position, temperature, shape and size, mucosal integrity, and discharge.

8. Pain noted while palpating the patient's cervical area may be an indication of inflammation of the uterus, ovaries, fallopian tubes, ligaments of the uterus, or inferior vena cava.

9. Rectovaginal palpation helps to assess the rectum, the posterior part of the uterus, the ovaries, and the pelvic cavity.

10. A bimanual examination is used to palpate the uterus, ovaries, and mons pubis.

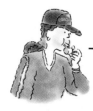

Coaching session

Pubic hair development

Pubic hair changes in density, color, and texture throughout a woman's life. Before adolescence, the pubic area is covered only with body hair. In adolescence, this body hair grows thicker, darker, coarser, and curlier. In full maturity, it spreads over the symphysis pubis and inner thighs. In later years, the hair grows thin, gray, and brittle.

■ You make the call

Identify which assessment procedure the nurse is performing, and briefly describe each step shown.

Assessment procedure: _____

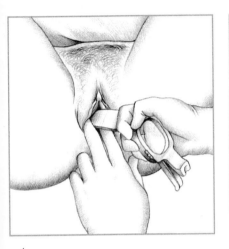 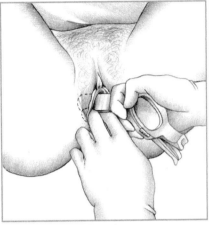 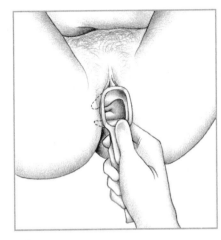

1. _____

_____

_____

2. _____

_____

_____

3. _____

_____

_____

■ Hit or miss

Indicate whether the following statements about internal genitalia examinations are true or false.

_____ 1. Nurses don't routinely inspect internal genitalia unless they're in advanced practice.

_____ 2. Only a water-soluble lubricant may be used to insert a vaginal speculum.

_____ 3. To palpate the cervix, sweep your fingers from side to side across the cervix and around the os.

_____ 4. To perform a rectovaginal examination, put on a new pair of gloves, apply a water-soluble lubricant to your index and middle fingers, ask the patient to bear down, then insert your index finger a short way into the vagina and your middle finger into her rectum.

True or false...A nurse can easily maintain her balance, poise, and concentration while reading a book and pedaling 25 laps around a workout course?

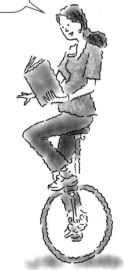

You make the call

There's nothing abnormal or tricky about these illustrations of the cervical os. Prove you're an assessment ace by correctly identifying what they depict.

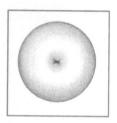

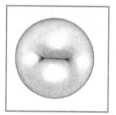

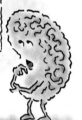

1. _____

2. _____

Match point

Match the bimanual examination technique in column 2 with its corresponding illustration in column 1.

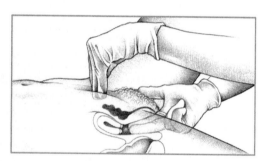

1. _____

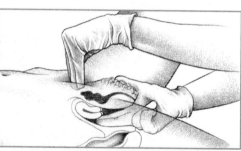

2. _____

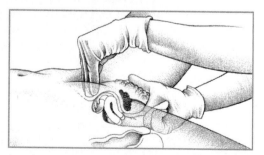

3. _____

Bimanual examination technique

A. Palpating the ovaries

B. Elevating the cervix and grasping the uterus

C. Palpating the posterior fornix and lower portion of the uterine wall

Cross-training

Here's a crossword puzzle to pump your brain cells and show off your ability to recognize abnormal genitourinary assessment findings.

Across

1. Absence of menstrual flow

3. Pain during urination that commonly signals a lower UTI

6. Herniation of rectum that appears as a pouch or bulging on posterior vaginal wall when patient bears down

7. STD caused by human papillomavirus that produces painless lesions on vulva, vagina, cervix, or anus (2 words)

9. Mild to severe cramping or colicky pain during menstruation

12. Infection that produces profuse, white, curdlike discharge with a yeasty odor

13. Presence of blood in urine

14. Excessive urination at night that's a common adverse effect of diuretics

15. Production and excretion of more than 2,500 ml of urine daily

16. Cramping pain at beginning of menstrual flow, abdominal bloating, breast tenderness, irritability, headache, and diarrhea (abbrev.)

17. Vaginal redness, itching, and discharge caused by overgrowth of an infectious organism

Down

2. Abnormal growth of uterine tissue

4. Unintentional passage of urine sometimes due to stress or a more serious problem

5. Infection that causes yellow, mucopurulent, odorless discharge, dysuria, and vaginal bleeding after douching or coitus

8. Vaginal prolapse

10. Symptoms include urinary urgency, hematuria, bladder spasms, and burning during urination (abbrev.)

11. Difficulty starting a urine stream

12. Bladder infection often accompanied by urinary frequency, straining to void, hematuria, perineal or lower-back pain, and low-grade fever

Match point

Now here's an easy exercise to help cool you down. Match the disorder in column 1 with the genitourinary findings in column 2.

Disorder

1. Early syphilis _____
2. Diabetic neuropathy _____
3. Urinary system obstruction _____
4. Gonorrhea _____
5. Bladder cancer _____

Genitourinary findings

A. Overflow incontinence and painless bladder distention

B. Dysuria throughout voiding, bladder distention, diminished urinary stream, urinary frequency and urgency, and sensation of bloating or fullness in lower abdomen or groin

C. Urge or overflow incontinence, hematuria, dysuria, nocturia, urinary frequency, suprapubic pain from bladder spasms, and palpable mass on bimanual examination

D. Chancrous red, painless, eroding lesion with a raised, indurated border that usually appears inside the vagina

E. Yellow or green, foul-smelling discharge that can be expressed from Bartholin's or Skene's ducts; dysuria; urinary frequency and incontinence; vaginal redness and swelling

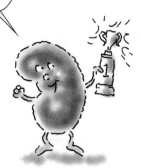

You've made it through another chapter…Well done! Now have a tall glass of water on me!

11

Male genitourinary system

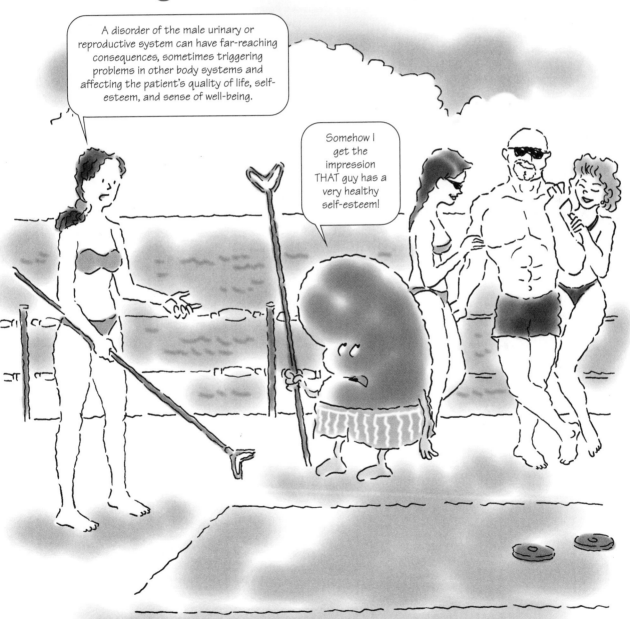

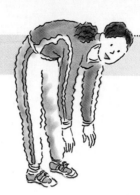
Male genitourinary system review

Genitourinary structures

◾ Urinary structures: similar to those in the female genitourinary system, including kidneys, ureters, bladder, and urethra; extra 6″ (15.2 cm) in male urethra to pass through the penis

◾ Penis: consists of the shaft, glans, urethral meatus, corona, and prepuce (foreskin); discharges urine as well as sperm

◾ Scrotum: loose, wrinkled sac that contains the testicles, epididymides, and portions of the spermatic cords

◾ Testicles: oval, rubbery structures that produce testosterone and sperm

◾ Epididymis: reservoir for mature sperm located on the posterolateral surface of each testicle

◾ Vas deferens: storage site and pathway for sperm

◾ Seminal vesicles: saclike glands found on the lower posterior surface of the bladder whose secretions help form seminal fluid

◾ Prostate gland: produces a thin, milky fluid that mixes with seminal fluid to enhance sperm activity

The health history

◾ Determine the patient's chief complaint.
  – Common urinary problems include pain on urination and changes in voiding pattern or urine color or output.
  – Common reproductive problems include penile discharge, erectile dysfunction, infertility, scrotal or inguinal masses, and pain or tenderness.

◾ Ask about past health and family health, especially about the presence or history of diabetes or hypertension.

◾ Ask about current health, such as circumcision status; penile sores, lumps, ulcers, or discharge; and scrotal swelling.

◾ Ask about sexual health and practices, including any history of sexually transmitted diseases and performance of testicular self-examination.

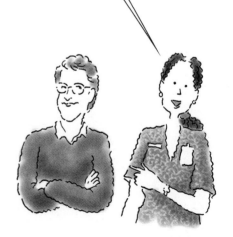

Keep in mind that a personal or family history of diabetes or hypertension can seriously affect your patient's genitourinary health.

Assessment

Urinary system

▪ Inspect the patient's skin and abdomen.
▪ Percuss and palpate the kidneys and bladder.
▪ Auscultate the renal arteries to check for bruits.

Reproductive system

▪ Inspect the penis for size, skin color, and abnormalities; compress the tip of the glans to inspect the urethral meatus.
▪ Inspect the scrotum, testicles, and pubic hair.
▪ Inspect the inguinal and femoral areas for bulges or hernias.
▪ Palpate the entire penile shaft.
▪ Gently palpate both testicles, assessing their size, shape, and response to pressure; transilluminate hard, irregular areas or lumps.
▪ Palpate the epididymides and both spermatic cords.
▪ Palpate for direct and indirect inguinal and femoral hernias.
▪ Palpate the prostate gland by performing a rectal examination.

Abnormal findings

Urinary system

▪ Hematuria: presence of blood in urine
▪ Urinary frequency: abnormally frequent urination
▪ Urinary urgency: intense and immediate desire to urinate
▪ Urinary hesitancy: hesitancy in starting urine stream
▪ Nocturia: excessive urination at night

Reproductive system

▪ Paraphimosis: tight prepuce that, when retracted, gets caught behind the glans and can't be replaced
▪ Hypospadias: urethral meatus located on the underside of the penis
▪ Epispadias: urethral meatus located on top of the penis
▪ Hydrocele: collection of fluid in the testicle
▪ Hernia: protrusion of an organ through a muscle wall
▪ Erectile dysfunction: inability to achieve and maintain penile erection sufficient to complete satisfactory sexual intercourse
▪ Priapism: persistent, painful erection unrelated to sexual excitation

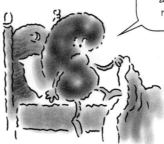

Always ask about problems with urination, such as urgency and excessive urination at night, which reminds me...

■■ ■ Hit or miss

Some of the following statements about the male genitourinary system are true; others are false. Mark each accordingly.

_____ 1. Urine formation and regulation of fluid and electrolyte balance occur in the highly vascular kidneys.

_____ 2. The urinary system helps maintain homeostasis by regulating fluid and electrolyte balance and producing the hormones erythropoietin and testosterone.

_____ 3. Major urinary system organs include the ureters, which attach to the kidneys and drain urine; the bladder, which lies directly behind the symphysis pubis and collects urine; and the urethra, which passes urine to outside the body.

_____ 4. The prostate is a fleshy, erectile organ consisting of the shaft, glans, urethral meatus, corona, and prepuce.

_____ 5. Semen is the only substance forcefully ejaculated from the urethral meatus during sexual activity.

_____ 6. Located below the penis, the scrotum includes two compartments, each housing an epididymis, portions of the spermatic cord, and a testicle.

_____ 7. Maturing sperm are stored in the vas deferens, a reservoir-like structure attached to the testicle's surface.

_____ 8. Testosterone stimulates changes that occur during puberty, which starts between ages 9½ and 13½.

_____ 9. The prepuce, also known as _foreskin,_ is sometimes removed after birth by circumcision.

_____ 10. The male urethra is considered a part of both the urinary system and reproductive system because it carries semen as well as urine.

_____ 11. The prostate gland produces a thin, milky, alkaline fluid that mixes with seminal fluid during ejaculation to enhance sperm activity.

_____ 12. The male urethra is typically shorter than the female urethra.

_____ 13. Testicular enlargement is typically the first sign of pubertal changes in males.

_____ 14. The right side of the scrotum is typically longer than the left.

_____ 15. Development of male secondary sex characteristics includes pubic hair growth and an increase in penis size.

> You'd think this would be easy with all that testosterone flowing through my body!

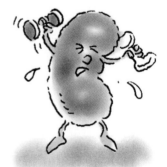

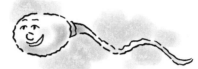

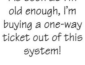

Finish line

Identify the major structures of the male genitourinary system in this illustration.

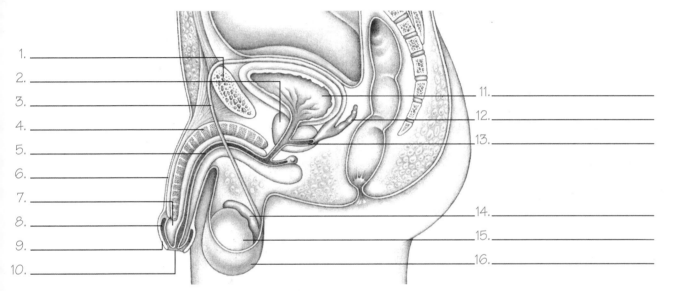

1. _____

2. _____

3. _____

4. _____

5. _____

6. _____

7. _____

8. _____

9. _____

10. _____

11. _____

12. _____

13. _____

14. _____

15. _____

16. _____

Brain crunches

Think fast! What are the four most common complaints about the reproductive system reported during a patient's health history?

1. _____

2. _____

3. _____

4. _____

▪▪ Strikeout

Stay in the game by correctly crossing out the term or phrase that doesn't belong in these statements about male genitourinary assessment.

1. Sores, lumps, ulcers, or absence of hair on the penis can signal a sexually transmitted disease.

2. During the health assessment, it's important to ask about the patient's history of diabetes, kidney stones, bladder infections, hypotension, and catheterization.

3. Scrotal swelling can be a sign of hiatal hernia, inguinal hernia, hematocele, epididymitis, or testicular cancer.

4. To assess sexual risk-taking behaviors, it's appropriate to ask about a patient's sexual preference, circumcision status, usual sexual practices, HIV status, and birth control measures.

5. Factors that can raise the scrotal temperature and temporarily diminish a patient's sperm count include frequent bicycle or motorcycle riding, taking hot baths, using an athletic supporter, and wearing boxer shorts.

> Get ready..."Ur-ine" for a challenging workout with this exercise!

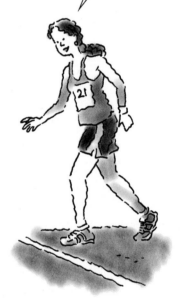

▪▪ Match point

Get a leg up on your patient's urinary health by asking about any noticeable urine changes. Match the urine color change in column 1 with the possible cause in column 2.

Urine color change

1. Pale and diluted _____

2. Orange-red or orange-brown _____

3. Blue-green _____

4. Dark yellow or amber and concentrated _____

5. Green-brown _____

6. Dark brown or black _____

7. Red or red-brown _____

Possible cause

A. Methylene blue ingestion

B. Acute glomerulonephritis, intake of chlorpromazine

C. Diabetes insipidus, diuretic therapy, excessive fluid intake

D. Bile duct obstruction

E. Hemorrhage, porphyria, intake of phenazopyridine

F. Obstructive jaundice, urobilinuria, intake of rifampin or phenazopyridine

G. Acute febrile disease, inadequate fluid intake, severe diarrhea or vomiting

You make the call

Identify the assessment techniques shown in the following illustrations, and briefly describe how they're done.

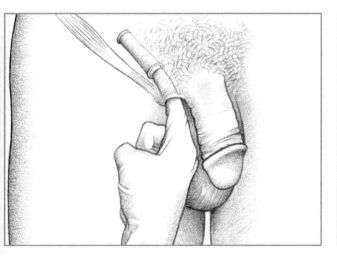

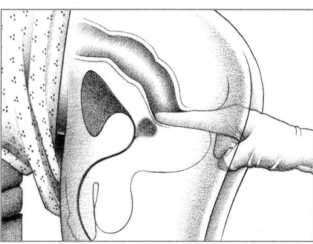

1. _____

_____

_____

_____

2. _____

_____

_____

_____

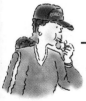

Coaching session
Teaching testicular self-examination

During your assessment, ask the patient whether he performs monthly testicular self-examinations. If he doesn't, explain that testicular cancer is the most common cancer in men ages 20 to 35 and that it can be treated successfully if detected early.

Teaching the technique
To do this examination, the patient should hold his penis out of the way with one hand, then roll each testicle between the thumb and first two fingers of his other hand. A normal testicle should have no lumps, move freely in the scrotal sac, and feel firm, smooth, and rubbery. Both testicles should be the same size, although the left one is usually lower than the right because the left spermatic cord is longer. Be sure to instruct the patient to notify his practitioner immediately if he finds any abnormalities.

Encourage your patient to perform monthly testicular self-examinations, and reinforce that he's an important player on the health care team. Go team!

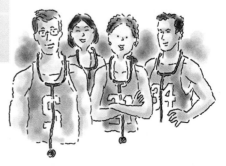

Cross-training

Exercise your mind and strengthen your vocabulary by working the clues to this crossword puzzle on male genitourinary assessment.

Across

4. Inability to replace the prepuce after it's retracted

9. Using a flashlight to examine testicle for abnormalities

11. Snowlike crystals on the skin from metabolic wastes (2 words)

12. Cheesy secretion commonly found beneath the prepuce

Down

1. Edema, increased urine protein levels, and decreased serum albumin levels (2 words)

2. Persistent, painful erection that's unrelated to sexual excitation

3. Smooth, moveable cord inside the spermatic cord that can be easily palpated (2 words)

5. Firm, white to yellow, nontender cutaneous lesions on scrotum or testicles (2 words)

6. Enlargement of this organ is classified from grade 1 to grade 4

7. Common name of tinea cruris (2 words)

8. Blood in the urine

10. Loop of bowel that protrudes through a muscle wall

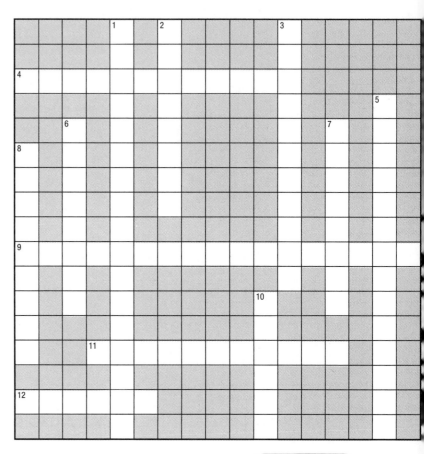

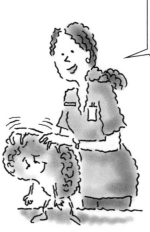

There's nothing like a good massage after exercising your brain with a challenging crossword puzzle.

Match point

Test your powers of observation by matching the genital lesion in column 2 with its corresponding illustration in column 1.

1. _____   2. _____   3. _____   4. _____

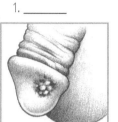 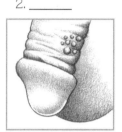 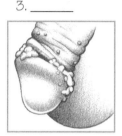 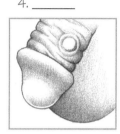

Genital lesion

A. Genital warts

B. Penile cancer

C. Syphilis

D. Genital herpes

Jumble gym

Unscramble the words below to discover terms related to abnormal male genitourinary assessment findings. Then use the circled letters to answer the question.

Question: Any one of these abnormal genitourinary findings can cause what reproductive problem?

1. R E L I C T E E   C O U N T Y F I N D S
   _ _ _ _ ◯ _ _   _ _ _ ◯ _ _ _ _ _ _

2. C H O R E D E L Y   _ _ _ _ _ _ ◯◯ _

3. G E N N I B   A C T O R P I T S   A H A S L I P P E R Y
   _ _ _ _ _ ◯ _   _ _ _ _ ◯ _ _ _   _ _ _ _ _ _ _ _ _ ◯ _

4. H A P P Y S O I D S A   _ ◯ _ _ _ _ _ _ _ _

5. P A S S I D E A P I   _ _ ◯ _ _ _ _ _ _ _

6. S A U C E R T I L T   U M R O T
   ◯ _ _ _ _ _ _ _ _ ◯ _   _ _ _ _ _

Answer: _ _ _ _ _ _ _ _ _ _ _

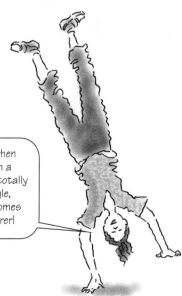

Sometimes, when you approach a problem from a totally different angle, everything becomes suddenly clearer!

Hit or miss

Indicate whether the following statements about assessment of the male genitourinary system are true or false.

_____ 1. Dullness percussed over the bladder may indicate retained urine in the bladder from bladder dysfunction or infection.

_____ 2. An enlarged scrotum in a boy younger than age 2 may be due to an inguinal hernia or a hydrocele, which is common in children of this age-group.

_____ 3. Hypospadias and epispadias are caused by traumatic injury to the penis and can lead to infertility.

_____ 4. A profuse, yellow discharge from the penis, possibly accompanied by urinary frequency, burning, and urgency, may be caused by syphilis.

_____ 5. Priapism is considered a urologic emergency because lack of prompt treatment can cause penile ischemia and thrombosis.

Team colors

Use a red pencil to trace the pathway of sperm through the genitourinary system, beginning with its formation and eventual ejaculation from the body.

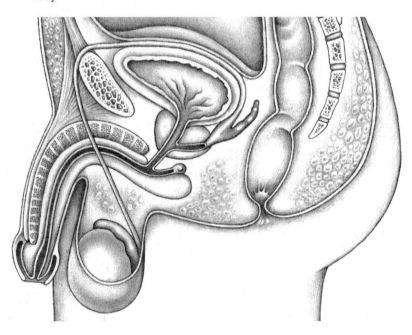

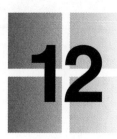

Musculoskeletal system

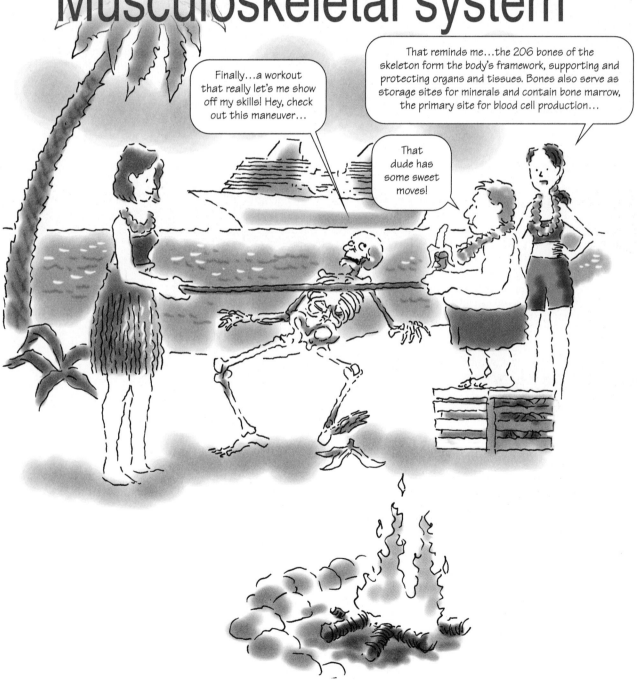

■■ ■ Warm-up

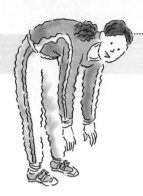

Musculoskeletal system review

Structures

Bones

- Support and protect organs and tissues
- Serve as storage sites for minerals
- Produce blood cells in bone marrow

Joints

- Defined as the junction of two or more bones
- Consist of two types
  - Nonsynovial: immovable or slightly movable bones connected by fibrous tissue or cartilage (such as the skull and vertebrae)
  - Synovial: freely movable bones that meet in a cavity filled with synovial fluid (a lubricant); include ball-and-socket and hinge joints
- Perform different types of motion
  - Circumduction: moving in a circular manner
  - Flexion: bending, decreasing the joint angle
  - Extension: straightening, increasing the joint angle
  - Abduction: moving away from midline
  - Adduction: moving toward midline
  - Retraction and protraction: moving backward and forward
  - Pronation: turning downward
  - Supination: turning upward
  - Internal rotation: turning toward midline
  - External rotation: turning away from midline
  - Eversion: turning outward
  - Inversion: turning inward

Muscles

- Consist of groups of contractile cells or fibers
- Attach to bone by tendons (tough fibrous portions of muscle)

The health history

- Determine the patient's chief complaint, such as pain, swelling, stiffness, and obvious deformities.
- Ask about current health, such as effects on activities of daily living and the use of ice, heat, or other remedies to treat the problem.
- Ask about past health, including arthritis, cancer, osteoporosis, and trauma, and inquire about the patient's use of assistive devices, such as a walker or cane.
- Ask about medications, especially those that may affect the musculoskeletal system (such as corticosteroids and potassium-depleting diuretics).
- Ask about lifestyle, including the patient's job, hobbies, and personal habits.

Assessing the musculoskeletal system

- Work from head to toe and from proximal to distal.
- Note the size and shape of joints, limbs, and body regions.
- Inspect and palpate around joints, limbs, and body regions.
- Have the patient perform active range-of-motion (ROM) exercises; if he can't, perform passive ROM exercises. Never force any movement.
- Observe the patient's posture and gait whenever possible.

Assessing bones and joints

Head, jaw, and neck

- Inspect the patient's face.
- Evaluate ROM in the temporomandibular joint.
- Inspect the front, back, and sides of the patient's neck.
- Palpate the cervical vertebrae and the neck area. Listen for crepitus as the patient moves his neck.
- Assess ROM in the neck.

Spine

- Inspect the patient's spine posteriorly and as he stands in profile.
- Assess for scoliosis by having the patient bend at the waist.
- Assess the range of spinal movement.
- Palpate the spinal processes and areas lateral to the spine as the patient bends at the waist.

Shoulders and elbows

- Inspect and palpate the shoulders.
- Assess internal and external rotation, flexion and extension, and abduction and adduction of the shoulders.
- Assess flexion and extension and supination and pronation of the elbows.

Wrists and hands

- Inspect and palpate the wrists and hands. Also palpate each finger joint.
- Assess ROM in the wrist: rotation, flexion, and extension. Assess for carpal tunnel syndrome if these movements cause pain or numbness.
- Assess extension and flexion of the metacarpophalangeal joints.
- Assess flexion, extension, abduction, and adduction of all the fingers.
- Measure both arms if you suspect one is longer than the other.

Hips and knees

- Inspect the hip area and knees.
- Palpate the hips and knees.
- Perform the bulge sign to assess for excess fluid in the knee joint.
- Assess hip flexion, extension, abduction, and adduction as well as internal and external hip rotation.
- Assess flexion and extension in the knee.

Ankles and feet

- Inspect and palpate the ankles and feet.
- Assess dorsiflexion, plantar flexion, inversion, and eversion of the ankles.
- Assess the metatarsophalangeal joints by having the patient flex and extend his toes.
- Measure both legs if you suspect one is longer than the other.

Assessment of the muscles

- Assess muscle tone as you move each limb through passive ROM exercises.
- Assess shoulder, arm, wrist, and hand strength.
- Assess leg strength.

Abnormal musculoskeletal findings

- Crepitus: abnormal crunching or grating that may be heard or felt when a joint with roughened articular surfaces moves
- Footdrop: plantar flexion of the foot with the toes bent toward the instep
- Heberden's nodes: hard nodes on the distal interphalangeal joints in patients with osteoarthritis
- Bouchard's nodes: hard nodes on the proximal interphalangeal joints in patients with osteoarthritis
- Muscle atrophy: muscle wasting
- Muscle spasms: muscle cramps; strong, painful muscle contractions

The 5 P's of musculoskeletal injury

- Pain
- Paresthesia
- Paralysis
- Pallor
- Pulse

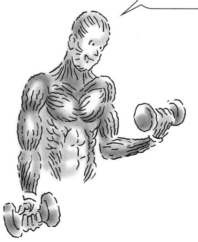

Don't forget to check out your patient's muscles when performing a musculoskeletal assessment. What do you think of these biceps?

■ Batter's box

Fill in the blanks and bone up on your knowledge of musculoskeletal anatomy and physiology.

Oh, them bones!

The human skeleton contains _____ bones, forming the body's frame-
1

work and supporting and protecting _____ and _____ .
2   3

Bones serve as a storage site for minerals and contain _____ , the pri-
4

mary site for blood cell production. _____ are junctures where two or
5

more bones meet; they stabilize bones and allow a specific type of

_____ . There are two types of joints: _____ joints, in
6   7

which bones are connected by fibrous tissue or cartilage, allowing little or no move-

ment, and _____ joints, in which cartilage-lined bones meet in a fluid-
8

filled cavity that allows the bones to move freely. _____ are tough, fi-
9

brous bands that join one bone to another. Common examples of synovial joints in-

clude _____ joints, such as the shoulders and hips, and
10

_____ joints, such as the knee and elbow.
11

Muscle-up

Muscles are groups of _____ cells or fibers that effect movement of an
12

organ or a part of the body. _____ are tough fibrous portions of muscle that at-
13

tach muscles to bone. _____ are sacs filled with friction-reducing syn-
14

ovial fluid that allow adjacent muscles or muscles and tendons to glide smoothly

over each other during movement. _____ is a smooth, fibrous tissue
15

that cushions the end of each bone. _____ fills the space between
16

joints, lubricating the joints and easing movement.

Options

ball-and-socket

bone marrow

bursae

cartilage

contractile

hinge

joints

ligaments

movement

nonsynovial

organs

synovial

synovial fluid

tendons

tissues

206

Who ordered the ribs? Bone appétit!

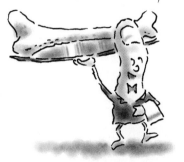

■ Team up!

Now let's see how well you can classify your bones. Write each bone type under its appropriate skeletal classification.

Axial skeleton

_____

_____

_____

_____

_____

_____

_____

Appendicular skeleton

_____

_____

_____

_____

_____

_____

_____

Bones
- Hyoid
- Shoulders
- Legs
- Sternum
- Skull
- Pelvis
- Arms
- Ribs
- Facial bones
- Vertebrae

■ Finish line

Identify the major structures of a synovial joint as shown in this illustration.

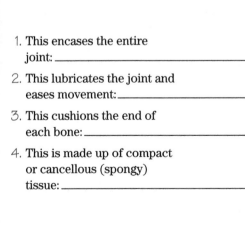

1. This encases the entire joint: _____

2. This lubricates the joint and eases movement: _____

3. This cushions the end of each bone: _____

4. This is made up of compact or cancellous (spongy) tissue: _____

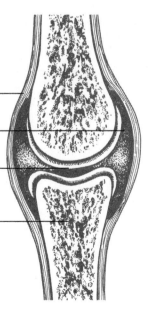

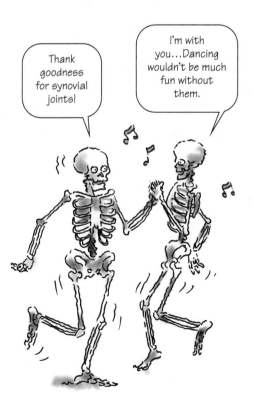

Thank goodness for synovial joints!

I'm with you...Dancing wouldn't be much fun without them.

Finish line

Have we got a bone to pick with you! See if you can identify all 30 bones shown in these illustrations.

Someone mentioned there'd be skeletons and games in this chapter so, naturally, I thought 'Halloween party.' Must have gotten my signals crossed!

Anterior view

1. _____
2. _____
3. _____
4. _____
5. _____
6. _____
7. _____
8. _____
9. _____
10. _____
11. _____
12. _____
13. _____
14. _____
15. _____

16. _____
17. _____
18. _____

Posterior view

1. _____
2. _____
3. _____
4. _____
5. _____
6. _____
7. _____
8. _____
9. _____
10. _____
11. _____
12. _____

Match point

Exercising is easy when you have all the right moves. Match each term with its corresponding body movement description and illustration.

1. Moving in a circular manner _____

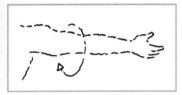

2. Bending, decreasing the joint angle _____

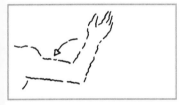

3. Straightening, increasing the joint angle _____

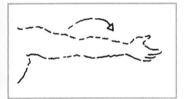

4. Moving away from midline _____

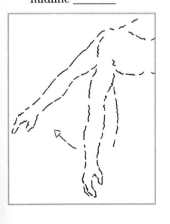

5. Moving backward and forward _____

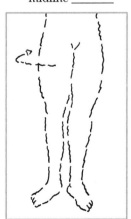

6. Turning downward _____

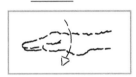

7. Turning upward _____

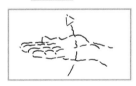

8. Moving toward midline _____

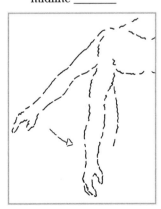

9. Turing toward midline _____

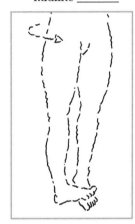

10. Turing away from midline _____

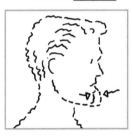

11. Turning outward _____

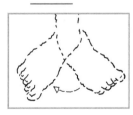

12. Turning inward _____

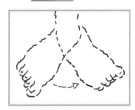

Term

A. Internal rotation

B. Abduction

C. Extension

D. Pronation

E. Inversion

F. Supination

G. Circumduction

H. Adduction

I. Eversion

J. External rotation

K. Retraction and protraction

L. Flexion

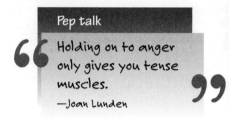

■ Jumble gym

Unscramble the words below to discover terms related to musculoskeletal signs and symptoms. Then use the circled letters to answer the question.

Question: **You may not have time for a thorough patient assessment because many musculoskeletal injuries present as what?**

1. N A P I   _ _ _ ◯

2. L E G S N I L W   _ _ ◯ _ _ _ _ ◯

3. S N I T S E F F S   _ _ ◯ _ _ _ ◯ _ _

4. T I D Y M E R O F   _ _ _ _ _ ◯ _ _ _

5. S E E S W A N K   _ _ _ _ _ ◯ _ _

6. S H I N E S A C   _ ◯ _ _ _ _ ◯ _

7. F U R C R A T E   _ ◯ _ _ _ _ _ ◯

Answer: _ _ _ _ _ _ _ _ _ _

■ Brain crunches

Just when you thought you were through taking history tests…Answer this question correctly and you'll have one dandy checklist to keep on hand for musculoskeletal system assessments.

Question: **Focusing on which seven factors during the health history can provide helpful clues about your patient's musculoskeletal injury or problem?**

1. _____
2. _____
3. _____
4. _____
5. _____
6. _____
7. _____

I'm fishing for seven answers here!

Hit or miss

Indicate whether the following statements about musculoskeletal system assessment are true or false.

_____ 1. Because the cardiovascular system and musculoskeletal system are interrelated, you should assess them together.

_____ 2. Use inspection, palpation, and auscultation to assess all bones, joints, and muscles.

_____ 3. Perform an abbreviated assessment if the patient has pain in only one body area; otherwise, perform a complete assessment if he has generalized symptoms.

_____ 4. Passive range-of-motion exercises require the patient to exert only minimal effort.

_____ 5. A person who walks normally will have a torso that sways only slightly, arms that swing naturally at his sides, an even gait, and erect posture.

_____ 6. A waddling, ducklike gait in a child is an important indicator of hypocalcemia.

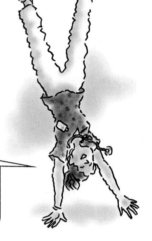

There's nothing like a true-or-false quiz to limber up your mind and fire off some neurons!

You make the call

Identify the musculoskeletal sign being evaluated in this illustration; then briefly explain its clinical significance.

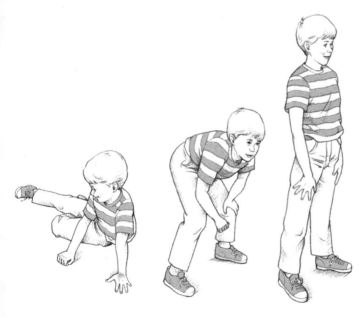

Answer: _____

_____

_____

_____

_____

_____

_____

_____

In the ballpark

Indicate the normal range of motion by circling the correct response in the middle column.

Assessment area	Normal ROM	Direction or movement
Neck	30° 40° 50°	Touching each ear to each shoulder
	25° 35° 45°	Forward flexion
	55° 65° 75°	Backward extension
Shoulder	90° 125° 180°	Flexion
	15° 45° 90°	Extension
Wrist	25° 55° 80°	Lateral rotation
	20° 30° 50°	Medial rotation
Hip	35° 45° 55°	Abduction
	30° 40° 50°	Adduction
Knee	90° 100° 125°	Flexion
	0° 25° 45°	Extension
Foot	25° 35° 45°	Plantar flexion
	0° 20° 40°	Dorsiflexion

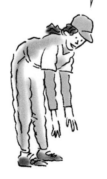
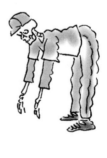

It may not be the 7th inning, but this seems like the perfect time to stretch.

Batter's box

Fill in the blanks with the appropriate terms related to physical assessment of the musculoskeletal system.

▪ If you hear or palpate a click as the patient's mouth opens, suspect an improperly

aligned jaw or _____ dysfunction.
₁

▪ _____ and _____ are examples of spinal curvature dis-
₂ ₃

orders.

▪ The length of the _____ from neck to waist usually increases by
₄

at least 2″ (5 cm) when a patient bends forward.

▪ Subcutaneous nodules palpated in the elbow or ulna may be a

sign of _____ .
₅

▪ The difference between the left and right extremities (for arms

and legs) should be no more than _____ inch.
₆

Options
⅜
kyphosis
lordosis
rheumatoid arthritis
spine
temporomandibular joint

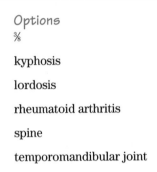

Coaching session
Testing for scoliosis

To test for scoliosis, first have the patient remove his shirt and stand as straight as possible with his back to you. Look for:
• uneven shoulder height and shoulder blade prominence
• unequal distance between the arms and body
• asymmetrical waistline
• uneven hip height
• sideways lean.

Bent over
Then have the patient bend forward, keeping his head down and palms together. Look for the following (pictured below):
• asymmetrical thoracic spine or prominent rib cage (rib hump) on either side
• asymmetrical waistline.

Winner's circle

Circle the picture that shows kyphosis, or abnormal curvature of the thoracic spine.

1.
2.

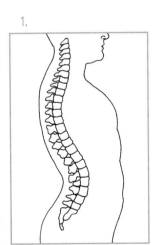
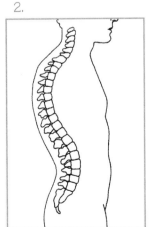

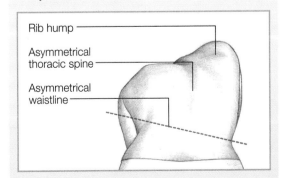

Rib hump

Asymmetrical thoracic spine

Asymmetrical waistline

■ You make the call

Identify the tests being performed in each illustration, and briefly describe how and why they're done.

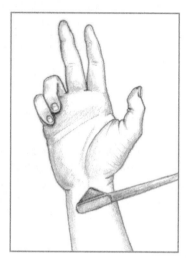

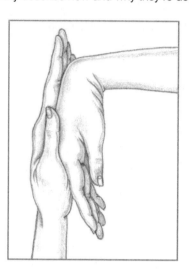

1. _____

_____

_____

_____

2. _____

_____

_____

_____

■ Brain crunches

List five types of traumatic injury affecting the musculoskeletal system—STAT!

1. _____

2. _____

3. _____

4. _____

5. _____

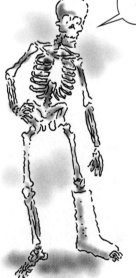

Careful...many traumatic injuries tend to occur when you're trying to get from here to there STAT!

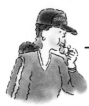

Coaching session
The 5 P's of assessing musculoskeletal injuries

To swiftly assess a musculoskeletal injury, remember the 5 P's: pain, paresthesia, paralysis, pallor, and pulse.

Pain
Ask the patient whether he feels pain. If he does, assess the location, severity, and quality of the pain.

Paresthesia
Assess the patient for loss of sensation by touching the injured area with the tip of an open safety pin. Abnormal sensation or loss of sensation indicates neurovascular involvement.

Paralysis
Assess whether the patient can move the affected area. If he can't, he might have nerve or tendon damage.

Pallor
Paleness, discoloration, and coolness on the injured side may indicate neurovascular compromise.

Pulse
Check all pulses distal to the injured site. If a pulse is decreased or absent, blood supply to the area is reduced.

■■ ■ You make the call

Identify the finding being assessed in these pictures, and then briefly describe the steps involved.

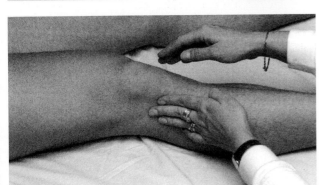

Assessment: _____

Steps

1. _____

_____

_____

_____

_____

2. _____

_____

_____

_____

_____

■ ■
■ Jumble gym

Unscramble the words below to discover terms related to musculoskeletal assessment.
Then use the circled letters to answer the question.

Question: **Assessment of what structures involves inspecting for tone, strength,
and symmetry as well as shortening and abnormal movement?**

1. P S M A S S   _ _ _ ◯ _ _

2. S T I C   _ _ ◯ _

3. C R O N E S C R A T U T   _ _ _ _ _ _ _ _ ◯ _ _ _

4. M E T S O R R   _ _ _ ◯ _ _ _

5. P H O R T Y Y E R P H   _ _ _ ◯ _ _ _ _ _ _

6. C L A S S I C F A T U O I N   _ _ ◯ _ _ _ _ ◯ _ _ _ _ _

Answer: _ _ _ _ _ _ _

■ ■
■ You make the call

Ow! Although these deformities may look painful, they're usually not.
Identify what they are and why they're clinically significant.

1. _____

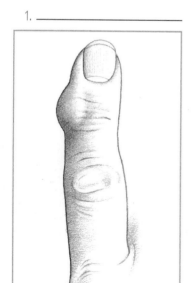

2. _____

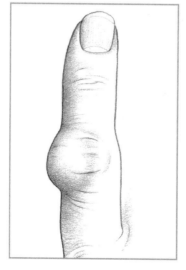

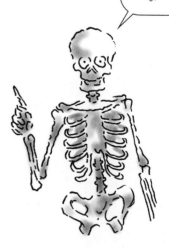

Make no bones
about it. Mental
workouts may be a little
painful, but like they
say, 'No pain, no gain.'

Clinical significance: _____

_____

Match point

Can you pass this muscle strength test? Match the muscle strength response in column 2 with the grade used in a typical muscle strength scale in column 1.

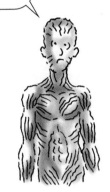

Gee...I hope they're grading on a curve!

Grade

1. 5/5 _____
2. 4/5 _____
3. 3/5 _____
4. 2/5 _____
5. 1/5 _____
6. 0/5 _____

Muscle strength response

A. Poor: Completes full ROM with gravity eliminated (passive motion)

B. Normal: Moves joint through full ROM and against gravity with full resistance

C. Trace: Attempt at muscle contraction is palpable but without joint movement

D. Good: Completes ROM against gravity with moderate resistance

E. Zero: No evidence of muscle contraction

F. Fair: Completes ROM against gravity only

You make the call

Identify the muscle strength testing techniques shown in the following illustrations.

1. _____

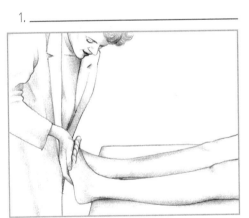

2. _____

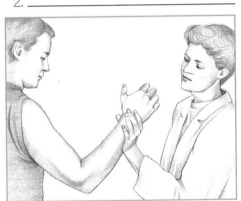

3. _____

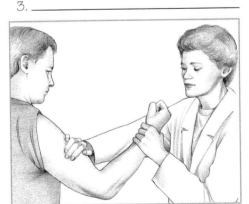

4. _____

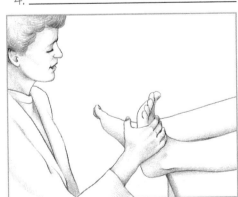

Cross-training

Complete this puzzle to test your knowledge of commonly encountered musculoskeletal problems.

Across

1. Muscle cramps
4. Inflammation of the fibrous portions of muscle that attach muscles to bone
6. Syndrome that causes pain, numbness, and tingling of the hand (2 words)
7. Out of alignment, as with a shoulder
8. Asymmetry of the thoracic spine and waistline with a noticeable rib hump
13. Abnormal rounding of the thoracic curve
14. Plantar flexion of the foot with the toes bent toward the instep

Down

2. Degenerative disease that causes progressive, irreversible skeletal muscle weakness
3. Having knees that point outward
4. A patient with an improperly aligned jaw may have dysfunction of this (abbrev.)
5. Having knees that turn inward
9. Abnormal grating sound sometimes heard in the neck
10. Abnormal curvature of the lumbar spine
11. Localized, painful swelling at the base of the great toe, often due to new bone growth or misalignment
12. To decrease in size or waste away

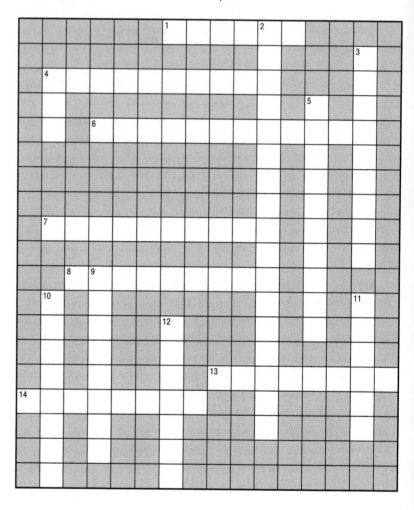

■ Train your brain

Sound out each group of pictures and symbols to reveal terms that complete this assessment consideration.

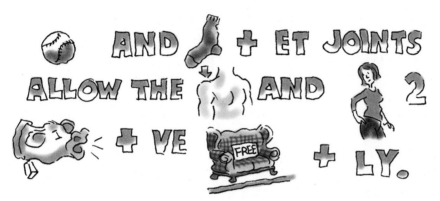

Answer: _____

■ Brain crunches

If you answer this question incorrectly, you may end up putting your foot in your mouth.

Can you list at least five common problems you might detect during a foot assessment?

1. _____
2. _____
3. _____
4. _____
5. _____

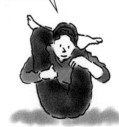

Strike out

Cross out the term or phrase that doesn't belong in these statements about abnormal musculoskeletal findings.

1. Painful and audible knee pops, inability to extend the leg fully, pronounced crepitus, a negative bulge sign, and sudden buckling are all considered abnormal.

2. Referred shoulder pain may be due to a dislocation, heart attack, or ruptured ectopic pregnancy.

3. Examples of spinal deformities include scoliosis, ecchymosis, kyphosis, and lordosis.

4. Temporomandibular joint dysfunction can lead to local swelling, crepitus, pain, sciatica, and lockjaw.

5. Hands should be carefully inspected for tenderness, maxillary edema, nodules, webbing between fingers, and boggy joints.

6. Corticosteroids can cause swelling, muscle weakness, myopathy, osteoporosis, pathologic fractures, and avascular necrosis of the heads of the femur and humerus.

7. Osteoporosis causes a decrease in bone mass that leaves bones porous, calcified, brittle, and prone to fracture.

8. Knitting, playing football or tennis, swimming, working at a computer, and doing construction work can cause repetitive stress injuries.

9. Muscle atrophy may result from neuromuscular disease or injury, metabolic and endocrine disorders, extensive exercising, prolonged immobility, or aging.

10. Muscle spasms commonly result from muscle fatigue, exercise, electrolyte imbalances, use of potassium-sparing diuretics, and pregnancy.

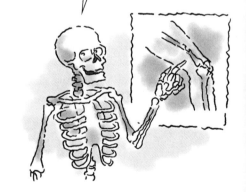

Finding a 'funny bone' here would definitely be abnormal—and, I might add, not a bit humerus!

■ Team up!

Here's a fun exercise...literally, a box of bones to sort out! Write each type of bone under its appropriate body location heading.

Upper extremities	Lower extremities	Torso
_____	_____	_____
_____	_____	_____
_____	_____	_____
_____	_____	_____
_____	_____	_____
_____	_____	_____
_____	_____	_____
_____	_____	_____
_____	_____	_____
_____	_____	_____
_____	_____	_____
_____	_____	_____
_____	_____	_____

Bones
- Acetabulum
- Acromion process
- Carpal
- Cervical vertebrae
- Clavicle
- Coccyx
- Femur
- Fibula
- Greater trochanter
- Humerus
- Iliac crest
- Ilium
- Ischium
- Lumbar vertebrae
- Metacarpal
- Metatarsals
- Patella
- Phalanges
- Radius
- Rib
- Scapula
- Sternum
- Tarsal
- Thoracic vertebrae
- Tibia
- Ulna

Pep talk

" Don't be discouraged by a failure. It can be a positive experience. Failure is, in a sense, the highway to success, inasmuch as every discovery of what is false leads us to seek earnestly after what is true, and every fresh experience points out some form of error which we shall afterwards carefully avoid. "

—John Keats

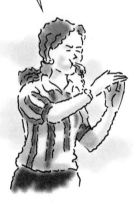

10-minute time-out
to review
musculoskeletal
system findings!

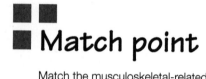

Match point

Match the musculoskeletal-related signs and symptoms in column 2 with the likely cause in column 1.

Signs and symptoms

1. Severe, localized pain that worsens with movement; ecchymosis and edema; deformity and crepitus; impaired circulation; muscle spasms _____

2. Shooting, aching, tingling pain that radiates down leg; pain exacerbated by activity and relieved by rest; limping; difficulty moving from a sitting to standing position _____

3. Muscle weakness, disuse, and possible atrophy; severe lower back pain, possibly radiating to buttocks, legs, and feet; diminished reflexes; sensory and personality changes; altered level of consciousness _____

4. Muscle weakness in one or more limbs, possibly leading to atrophy, spasticity, and contractures; hyperactive deep tendon reflexes; paresthesia or sensory loss; incoordination; intention tremors; diplopia, blurred vision, or vision loss _____

5. Discomfort ranging from calf tenderness to severe pain; edema and a feeling of heaviness in affected leg; warmth; fever, chills, malaise, and muscle cramps; positive Homans' sign _____

6. Tetany (muscle cramps and twitching, carpopedal and facial muscle spasms, and seizures); positive Chvostek's and Trousseau's signs; paresthesia of the lips, fingers, and toes; choreiform movements; hyperactive deep tendon reflexes; fatigue; palpitations and cardiac arrhythmias _____

7. Severe arm pain with passive muscle stretching; impaired distal circulation; muscle weakness; decreased reflex response; paresthesia; edema; possible paralysis and absent pulse _____

Likely cause

A. Sciatica

B. Multiple sclerosis

C. Hypocalcemia

D. Herniated disk

E. Compartment syndrome

F. Fracture

G. Thrombophlebitis

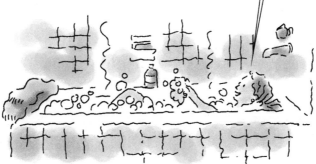

Answers

Chapter 1

Page 6

Batter's box

1. Patient history, 2. Physical examination, 3. Subjective,
4. Objective, 5. Communication, 6. Chief complaint,
7. Inspection, 8. Palpation, 9. Percussion, 10. Auscultation,
11. Nutrition, 12. Mental health, 13. Illness, 14. Treatment,
15. Behavior, 16. Coping, 17. Self-destructive behavior

Page 7

Team up!

Subjective data
- Headache
- Sore throat
- Tiredness
- Knee pain
- Anxiety
- Loss of taste
- Chest pain

Objective data
- Blood pressure: 131/82 mm Hg
- Respirations: 22 breaths/minute
- Cloudy urine
- Bleeding gums
- Tremors
- Dentures
- ECG results
- Weight loss of 15 lb
- Cough
- Eyeglasses
- Mottled skin
- Difficulty walking
- Temperature: 99.2°F

Page 8

Cross-training

■ Page 9

Finish line

1. Carotid, 2. Brachial, 3. Radial, 4. Femoral,
5. Popliteal, 6. Posterior tibial, 7. Pedal

Jumble gym

1. **numbness**
2. **shortness of breath**
3. **cramping**
4. **hair loss**
5. **itching**
6. **difficulty swallowing**
7. **twitching**
8. **headaches**
9. **chest pain**

Answer: chief complaint

■ Page 10

Mind sprints

Possible questions to ask:
- How would you describe your pain?
- Where does your pain occur?
- How frequently do you experience pain, and how long does it typically last?
- Do you feel any pain right now? Is it the same pain you usually feel, or is it different?
- How would you rate the pain on a scale of 0 to 10, with 0 being no pain and 10 being the worst pain imaginable?
- When did you first notice the pain? What were you doing at the time? Has it changed in any way since you first noticed it?
- What do you think causes the pain? Does anything seem to trigger or aggravate it?
- How has the pain affected your everyday life?
- What do you usually do to alleviate the pain? Any medications or other measures? Do they seem to relieve the pain?
- What are your expectations of the health care team in terms of managing your pain?

You make the call

1. Auscultation, 2. Palpation, 3. Percussion

■ Page 11

Match point

1. E, H; 2. D, J; 3. A, G; 4. C, I; 5. B; 6. F

■ Page 12

Obstacle course

1. Crowded, noisy office
2. Nurse is distracted; can't listen attentively; lack of eye contact with patient
3. Elderly patient, possibly with hearing or memory deficit
4. Possible language barrier
5. Possible cultural barrier

■ Page 13

Strikeout

1. Body temperature, pulse, respirations, ~~urine output~~, and blood pressure are part of a <u>vital signs</u> assessment.
2. Height, weight, head circumference, midarm circumference, skin-fold thickness, and ~~visual acuity~~ are considered <u>anthropometric</u> measurements.
3. Palpation, ~~mental assessment~~, auscultation, inspection, and percussion are <u>physical assessment</u> techniques.
4. ~~Urinary~~, oral, rectal, axillary, and tympanic are common methods of assessing <u>temperature</u>.
5. Color, size, location, movement, texture, ~~emotion~~, symmetry, odor, and sound are all assessed during the <u>physical inspection</u>.

Match point

1. C, 2. B, 3. F, 4. D, 5. A, 6. E

■ Page 14
Winner's circle

Triceps skin-fold

1.
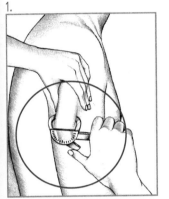

2.
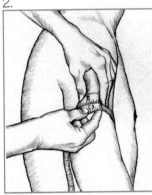

Midarm circumference

1.
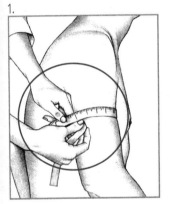

2.
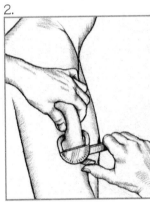

■ Page 15
Batter's box

1. Albumin, 2. Transferrin, 3. Triglycerides, 4. Hematocrit, 5. Nitrogen, 6. Cholesterol, 7. Hemoglobin

Mind sprints

Physical conditions
- Chronic illness (diabetes; neurologic, cardiac, or thyroid problems)
- Draining wounds, fistulas, burns
- Obesity, unplanned weight loss or gain
- Cystic fibrosis
- GI disturbances
- Anorexia, bulimia
- Depression, anxiety
- Severe trauma
- Chemotherapy, radiation therapy, bone marrow transplantation
- Paresis, paralysis, or other physical limitations
- Major surgery
- Pregnancy
- Mouth, tooth, denture problems

Drugs and diet
- Fad diets
- Steroids, diuretics, antacids
- Excessive alcohol intake
- Strict vegetarian diet
- Liquid diet

Sociocultural influences
- Lack of support
- Financial problems
- Religious observances
- Cultural, ethnic preferences
- Work schedule

■ Page 16
Match point

1. B, 2. G, 3. D, 4. F, 5. C, 6. E, 7. A, 8. H

■ Page 17

Jumble gym

1. rationalization
2. denial
3. fantasy
4. projection
5. repression
6. regression
7. displacement

Answer: Defense

Hit or miss

1. True, 2. True, 3. False (This describes *depersonalization*.), 4. False (Compulsions attempt to alleviate *obsessions*.), 5. True

■ Page 18

Three-point conversion

1. Echolalia
2. Clanging
3. Confabulation

■■ ■ Chapter 2

■ Page 22

Batter's box

1. Skin, 2. Organ, 3. Tissues, 4. Water, 5. Electrolytes, 6. Temperature, 7. Wound, 8. Dermis, 9. Epidermis, 10. Subcutaneous, 11. Keratin, 12. Follicle, 13. Papilla, 14. Melanocytes, 15. Lanugo, 16. Balding, 17. Genetically, 18. Keratin, 19. Cuticle, 20. Ridges

■ Page 23

Team up!

- Epidermis: Melanocyte, stratum germinativum, stratum corneum
- Dermis: Nerve, blood vessel, hair follicle, apocrine (sebaceous) gland, lymphatic vessel, eccrine (sweat) gland

Jumble gym

1. dry and flaky
2. pale color
3. tenting
4. wrinkling
5. parchmentlike

Answer: Old age

■ Page 24

Finish line

1. Epidermis, 2. Dermis, 3. Subcutaneous tissue, 4. Stratum corneum, 5. Pore of sweat gland, 6. Free nerve ending, 7. Eccrine sweat gland, 8. Hair bulb, 9. Sensory nerve fibers, 10. Autonomic nerve fibers, 11. Vein, 12. Artery

■ Page 25

Hit or miss

1. False (cells die off upon reaching surface), 2. False (not found in palms or soles), 3. True, 4. True, 5. False (they're called Mongolian spots), 6. True

You make the call

- Procedure: Evaluating skin turgor
- Assessment finding: Tenting, indicating poor turgor

■ Page 26

Finish line

1. Hair shaft, 2. Hair follicle, 3. Eccrine gland, 4. Apocrine gland, 5. Hair bulb, 6. Sebaceous duct, 7. Sebaceous gland, 8. Internal root sheath, 9. External root sheath, 10. Arrector pili muscle, 11. Matrix, 12. Hair papilla

Train your brain

Answer: Use a Wood's lamp to examine for fungal infections.

■ Page 27

Mind sprints

Possible questions
- What types of changes have you noticed (nail shape, color, brittleness)?
- When did you first notice changes in your nails?
- Were the changes gradual or sudden?
- Do you have any other signs or symptoms (bleeding, pain, itching, discharge)?
- What's the normal condition of your nails?
- Do you have any history of serious illness?
- Do you have a history of nail problems?
- Do you bite your nails or cuticles?
- Have you had nail tips attached?
- Have you ever experienced, or are you currently experiencing, stress, infection, or nutritional deficiencies?

Gear up!

- ☐ Bulb syringe
- ☑ Tongue blade
- ☑ Clear ruler (with mm and cm markings)
- ☑ Penlight, flashlight
- ☑ Wood's lamp
- ☐ Speculum
- ☐ Scale
- ☐ Percussion hammer
- ☐ Stethoscope
- ☑ Magnifying glass
- ☐ Otoscope
- ☐ Thermometer
- ☐ Tuning fork
- ☑ Gloves

■ Page 28

Match point

1. F, 2. C, 3. A, 4. G, 5. F, 6. B, 7. H, 8. D, 9. E, 10. I

■ Page 29

Choose the best course

| Assemble equipment, and put on gloves. |
| Observe skin's overall appearance. |
| Inspect and palpate skin, focusing on color, texture, turgor, moisture, and temperature. |
| Measure and note distribution of lesions. |
| Inspect and palpate hair, focusing on distribution, quantity, texture, and color. |
| Observe nail color, and press nail beds to assess peripheral circulation. |
| Inspect nail shape and contour, and palpate nail bed for thickness and strength. |

■ Page 30

Match point

1. C (early chickenpox), 2. A (freckle, flat nevus), 3. B (elevated nevus, wart)

■ Page 31

Team colors

   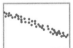

1. Discrete   2. Grouped   3. Confluent   4. Linear

5. Annular   6. Polycyclic   7. Arciform   8. Reticular

■ Page 32

Cross-training

	¹V	²I	T	I	L	I	G	O				
		M									³R	
		P									A	
⁴T	E	L	A	N	G	I	E	⁵C	T	A	S	I	A
		T						A			N	
		I						N			G	
		G			⁶U			D			W	
		O			R			I			O	
					T		⁷E	D		R		
					I		C	I		M		⁸L
					C		A	Z		E		U
⁹P	S	O	R	I	A	S	I	S		E		P
					R		I	M				U
					I		¹⁰S	C	A	B	I	E	S
					A							

■ Page 33

Finish line

1. Cuticle, 2. Nail bed, 3. Nail plate, 4. Lunula, 5. Matrix

You make the call

Assessment finding: Evaluating clubbed fingers
Significance: Good indicator of hypoxia, which is associated with pulmonary and cardiovascular conditions (emphysema, chronic bronchitis, lung cancer, heart failure)

■ Page 34

Three-point conversion

1. Hirsutism, 2. Diaphoresis, 3. Urticaria

■ Chapter 3

■ Page 39

Batter's box

1. Brain, 2. Spinal cord, 3. Cerebrum, 4. Lobes, 5. Hemispheres, 6. Midbrain, 7. Pons, 8. Medulla, 9. Reflex arc, 10. Nerves, 11. 12, 12. Motor, 13. Sensory, 14. Fight-or-flight, 15. Breathing

■ Page 40

Match point

1. C, 2. A, 3. B, 4. D

Strikeout

1. White matter, ~~blue matter~~, gray matter, posterior horn, and anterior horn are all part of the <u>spinal cord</u>.
2. Level of consciousness, appearance and behavior, ~~height and weight~~, speech, cognitive function, and constructional ability should be evaluated as part of a patient's <u>mental status</u>.
3. Facial nerve, oculomotor nerve, olfactory nerve, ~~radial nerve~~, and hypoglossal nerve are examples of <u>cranial</u> nerves.
4. ~~Babinski's~~, brachioradialis, triceps, and Achilles are <u>deep tendon</u> reflexes.

■ Page 41

Finish line

Brain
1. Cerebellum, 2. Cerebrum, 3. Thalamus, 4. Hypothalamus, 5. Midbrain, 6. Pituitary gland, 7. Pons, 8. Medulla, 9. Spinal cord

Spinal cord
1. Posterior horn, 2. Anterior horn, 3. White matter, 4. Gray matter

■ Page 42
Team colors

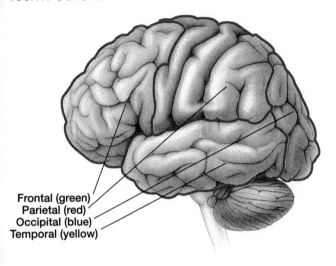

Frontal (green)
Parietal (red)
Occipital (blue)
Temporal (yellow)

■ Page 43
Train your brain

Answer: A simple reflex arc requires a sensory neuron and a motor neuron.

■ Page 44
You make the call

Answer: **Patellar reflex arc (knee-jerk reflex):** A sensory receptor detects a stimulus (reflex hammer striking patellar tendon), and the sensory neuron carries the impulse along its axon by way of the spinal nerve to the dorsal root ganglion, where it enters the spinal column. In the anterior horn of the spinal cord, the sensory neuron joins with a motor neuron, which carries the impulse along its axon by way of a spinal nerve to the muscle fibers through stimulation of the motor end plate, causing the muscle to contract and the leg to extend.

■ Page 45
Brain crunches

1. Headache, 2. Dizziness, 3. Faintness, 4. Confusion, 5. Impaired mental status, 6. Gait or balance disturbances, 7. Level of consciousness changes

Choose the best course

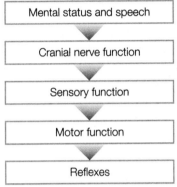

Mental status and speech

Cranial nerve function

Sensory function

Motor function

Reflexes

■ Page 46
Match point

1. D, 2. F, 3. I, 4. G, 5. H, 6. E, 7. B, 8. C, 9. A

Train your brain

Answer: An altered level of consciousness is the earliest sign of a changed neuro status.

■ Page 47

Team up!

Level of consciousness
- Lethargy
- Stuporousness
- Opens eyes when told to

Appearance and behavior
- Poor grooming
- Inappropriate clothes for season

Speech
- Dysarthria
- Use of clanging

Cognitive function
- Responds appropriately to hypothetical situation
- Confusion
- Poor attention span
- Memory loss
- Depression

Constructional ability
- Inability to button clothing when asked
- Holds pencil but can't draw square

Photo finish

1. **Decorticate posture:** Indicates abnormal flexion; Glasgow Coma Scale score of 3 for motor response
2. **Decerebrate posture:** Indicates abnormal extension; Glasgow Coma Score of 2 for motor response

■ Page 48

Hit or miss

1. True, 2. False (cranial nerves III, IV, and VI are tested together for this reason), 3. False (cranial nerve VIII is the acoustic nerve), 4. True, 5. True, 6. True, 7. False (they overlap in the pharynx), 8. True

■ Page 49

Match point

1. E, 2. B, 3. D, 4. C, 5. A

■ Page 50

Jumble gym

1. shoulder girdle
2. range of motion
3. muscle tone
4. Romberg's test
5. coordination
6. muscle strength

Answer: Cerebellum

Brain crunches

1. Ask patient to walk heel to toe, and observe his balance.
2. Ask patient to touch his nose, then your outstretched finger as you move it, repeating this motion faster and faster.
3. Ask patient to touch the thumb of his right hand to his right index finger and then each of his remaining fingers.
4. Ask patient to sit with palms on thighs and then to turn palms up and down, gradually increasing his speed.
5. Ask patient to alternately tap the soles of his feet against your palms while lying supine, gradually increasing his speed.

■ Page 51

You make the call

1. Brachioradialis, 2. Biceps, 3. Patellar, 4. Triceps, 5. Achilles

■ Page 52

Brain crunches

1. Altered level of consciousness, 2. Cranial nerve impairment, 3. Abnormal muscle movements, 4. Abnormal gaits

Match point

1. B, 2. E, 3. D, 4. A, 5. C

■ Page 53

Cross-training

¹T		²P							³B			
R		A						⁴G	R	A	S	P
I		T							A			
⁵C	R	E	M	⁶A	S	T	E	R	I	C		
E		L		C					H			
P		L		H			⁷B	I	C	E	P	⁸S
S		A		I					O			N
		R		L					R			O
		⁹G	L	A	B	E	L	L	A			U
				E					D			T
		¹⁰S	U	C	K				I			
									A			
¹¹A	B	D	O	M	I	N	A	L				
								I				
		¹²B	A	B	I	N	S	K	I			

■ Page 54

Team up!

Early signs
- Pupil changes on side of lesion
- Subtle orientation loss
- Sudden quietness
- Positive pronator drift (with palms up, one hand pronates)
- Sudden weakness
- Restlessness and anxiety
- Motor changes on side opposite lesion
- One pupil constricts but then dilates (unilateral hippus)
- Requires increased stimulation
- Intermittent increases in blood pressure
- Sluggish reaction of both pupils

Late signs
- Profound weakness
- Pupils fixed and dilated or "blown"
- Unarousable
- Increased systolic pressure, profound bradycardia, abnormal respirations (Cushing's triad)

■ Page 55

Hit or miss

1. True, 2. False (it's a form of expressive aphasia), 3. True, 4. False (this defines ideomotor apraxia), 5. True, 6. True, 7. True, 8. False (global aphasia is the lack of both receptive and expressive language; Wernicke's aphasia is a type of receptive aphasia), 9. True, 10. False (they're associated with lower motor neuron dysfunction)

■ Page 56

Winner's circle

1. Unilateral, dilated pupils

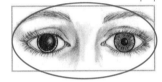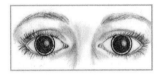

2. Bilateral pinpoint pupils

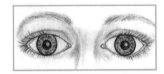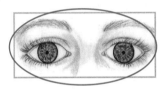

Chapter 4

Page 60

Batter's box

1. diabetic retinopathy, 2. cataracts, 3. elderly,
4. toxoplasmosis, 5. cytomegalovirus, 6. strabismus,
7. amblyopia, 8. eyelids, 9. lashes, 10. cornea, 11. iris, 12. retina,
13. muscles, 14. cranial nerves

Page 61

Match point

1. K, 2. J, 3. L, 4. I, 5. B, 6. G, 7. D, 8. A, 9. M, 10. F, 11. C,
12. E, 13. H

Page 62

Finish line

1. Choroid layer, 2. Central retinal artery and vein, 3. Optic
nerve, 4. Retina, 5. Ciliary body, 6. Sclera, 7. Vitreous humor,
8. Bulbar conjunctiva, 9. Schlemm's canal, 10. Cornea, 11. Lens,
12. Pupil, 13. Iris, 14. Anterior chamber, 15. Posterior chamber

Page 63

Brain crunches

1. Double vision (diplopia), 2. Visual floaters, 3. Photophobia
(light sensitivity), 4. Vision loss, 5. Eye pain

Mind sprints

Possible questions:
- Could you tell me about any problems you are having with your
eyes?
- Do you have a history of eye problems?
- Do you wear corrective lenses for distance or reading?
- Have you ever experienced blurred vision, blind spots, floaters,
double vision, discharge, or unusual sensitivity to light?
- How is your vision at night?
- Have you ever had an eye injury or eye surgery?
- Did you ever have a lazy eye?
- Do you have allergies?
- When was your last eye exam?
- Do you have eye pain or headaches?
- Do you squint to see objects at a distance?
- Do you have to hold objects close to, or far away from, your eyes
to see them?

Page 64

Gear up!

- ☐ Stethoscope
- ☑ Lamp or other light source
- ☑ Ophthalmoscope
- ☐ Speculum
- ☐ Scale
- ☐ Measuring tape
- ☐ Safety pin
- ☑ Vision test cards
- ☑ Gloves
- ☑ Cotton-tipped applicators
- ☐ Tongue blade
- ☑ Tissues
- ☑ Penlight
- ☑ Opaque cards
- ☐ Otoscope
- ☐ Povidone-iodine solution
- ☐ Syringe and needle

Page 65

Match point

1. E, 2. B, 3. D, 4. A, 5. C

You make the call

1. **Snellen alphabet chart:** used to test distance vision and
measure visual acuity in those who can read
2. **Snellen E chart:** used to test distance vision and measure
visual acuity in children and adults who can't read

Page 66

Three-point conversion

1. Assessing peripheral vision with confrontation, 2. Assessing
the six cardinal positions of gaze, 3. Assessing corneal sensitivity

■ Page 67

Hit or miss

1. False (these are good ways to evaluate extraocular muscles), 2. True, 3. True, 4. False (this is the red reflex), 5. False (this tests near vision), 6. True, 7. True, 8. False (arteries are thinner and brighter than veins)

Winner's circle

1.

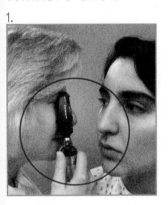

2.

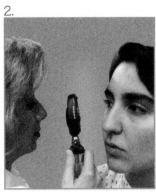

■ Page 68

Team colors

1. Superonasal arteriole and vein, 2. Superotemporal arteriole and vein, 3. Physiologic cup, 4. Optic disk, 5. Vein, 6. Arteriole, 7. Fovea centralis, 8. Macular area, 9. Inferonasal arteriole and vein, 10. Inferotemporal arteriole and vein

■ Page 69

Mind sprints

1. Bacterial conjunctivitis: purulent, unilateral greenish white discharge; sticky eyelid crusts that form during sleep; itching and burning; excessive tearing; sensation of foreign body in eye
2. Retinal detachment: sudden onset of spots or flashing lights; curtainlike loss of vision; black retinal vessels
3. Cataracts: gradual visual blurring; halo vision; visual glare in bright light; progressive vision loss; gray pupil that later turns milky white

You make the call

1. Periorbital edema, 2. Ptosis

■ Page 70

Match point

1. B, 2. H, 3. J, 4. C, 5. I, 6. G, 7. A, 8. E, 9. D, 10. F

■ ■ ■
■ Chapter 5

■ Page 74

Batter's box

1. cartilage, 2. pinna, 3. tympanic, 4. sound, 5. eustachian tube, 6. balance, 7. smell, 8. respiratory, 9. humidifying, 10. septum, 11. paranasal sinuses, 12. mucus, 13. nasopharynx, 14. oropharynx, 15. laryngopharynx, 16. palates, 17. tonsils, 18. neck, 19. thyroid, 20. triiodothyronine

■ Page 75

Cross-training

Crossword solution with the following filled answers: CRISTAE, THYROID, PHARYNX, KIESSELBACH, CARTILAGE, PARANASAL, VIBRATIONS, NARES, PERILYMPH, SEPTUM, and down entries including TYMPANIC, COCHLEA, SULCUS, MALLEUS, OLFACTORY, CURICLE, VULVA, UNA, LA.

■ Page 76

Finish line

1. External auditory canal, 2. Auricle (pinna), 3. Helix, 4. Anthelix, 5. Concha, 6. Antitragus, 7. Lobule, 8. Incus, 9. Malleus, 10. Tympanic membrane, 11. Footplate of stapes, 12. Vestibule, 13. Semicircular canals, 14. Cochlea, 15. Eustachian tube, 16. Acoustic nerve branches

■ Page 77

Brain crunches

1. Hearing loss, 2. Tinnitus (ringing in ears), 3. Pain, 4. Discharge, 5. Dizziness

Mind sprints

Possible questions:
■ Can you describe the problem with your ear, including when you first noticed it, where it occurs, and how long it typically lasts?
■ Does anything relieve or aggravate it?
■ Do you have any ear discharge? Can you describe the color and consistency?
■ Have you ever had a head injury?
■ Do you ever experience vertigo (spinning sensation)? When and how frequently do you have these episodes? Do you have nausea, vomiting, or tinnitus (ringing) when it occurs?
■ Have you ever had a previous ear problem or injury?
■ Does anyone in your family have ear problems?
■ Do you have any chronic illnesses? Have you been recently ill?
■ What medications do you currently take?
■ Do you have any allergies?

■ Page 78

You make the call

1. **Weber's test:** evaluates bone conduction; differentiates conductive hearing loss from sensorineural hearing loss
2. **Rinne test:** performed after Weber's test to compare air conduction of sound with bone conduction of sound; helps differentiate conductive hearing loss from sensorineural hearing loss

Hit or miss

1. True, 2. False (the opposite is true), 3. True, 4. False (he would have a sensorineural hearing loss), 5. True, 6. False (pull it up and back), 7. False (it should appear pearl gray, glistening, and transparent)

■ Page 79

Team colors

1. Pars flaccida, 2. Short process of malleus, 3. Handle of malleus, 4. Umbo, 5. Annulus, 6. Light reflex, 7. Pars tensa

Match point

1. C, 2. E, 3. A, 4. B, 5. D

■ Page 80

Finish line

1. Kiesselbach's area, 2. Superior turbinate, 3. Middle turbinate, 4. Inferior turbinate, 5. Adenoids, 6. Soft palate, 7. Hard palate, 8. Tongue, 9. Mandible, 10. Hard palate, 11. Soft palate, 12. Oropharynx, 13. Uvula, 14. Tongue, 15. Palatine tonsils

■ Page 81

You make the call

Palpation of maxillary sinuses: checks for tenderness; if tenderness is present, transillumination is performed to assess for fluid or pus or to reveal tumors and obstructions

Team colors

1. Preauricular, 2. Occipital, 3. Postauricular, 4. Anterior cervical, 5. Posterior cervical, 6. Supraclavicular, 7. Superficial cervical, 8. Tonsillar, 9. Submandibular, 10. Submental

■ Page 82

Batter's box

1. epistaxis, 2. ear, 3. esophageal, 4. nasal flaring, 5. laryngitis, 6. middle ear, 7. eardrum, 8. cerumen (ear wax), 9. sinuses, 10. cold

■■ ■ Chapter 6

■ Page 86

Batter's box

1. oxygenated, 2. waste products, 3. autonomic, 4. arteries, 5. veins, 6. blood pressure, 7. venae cavae, 8. aorta, 9. pericardium, 10. atria, 11. ventricles, 12. valves, 13. cardiac cycle, 14. sinoatrial, 15. systole, 16. diastole

■ Page 87

Match point

1. H, 2. F, 3. I, 4. C, 5. K, 6. E, 7. J, 8. A, 9. M, 10. L, 11. D, 12. G, 13. B

■ Page 88

Finish line

1. Superior vena cava, 2. Right atrium, 3. Right pulmonary veins, 4. Right ventricle, 5. Inferior vena cava, 6. Aortic arch, 7. Pulmonary artery, 8. Left pulmonary veins, 9. Left atrium, 10. Left ventricle, 11. Descending aorta

Page 89

Team colors

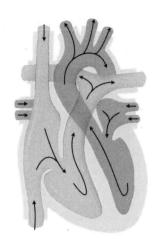

You make the call

1. **Diastole:** Phase of the cardiac cycle when the heart relaxes and the ventricles fill with blood
2. **Systole:** Phase of the cardiac cycle when the ventricles contract and blood is ejected into the pulmonary artery and the aorta

Page 90

Match point

1. B, 2. D, 3. A, 4. C

Brain crunches

1. Temporal artery, 2. Carotid artery, 3. Brachial artery, 4. Radial artery, 5. Ulnar artery, 6. Femoral artery, 7. Popliteal artery, 8. Posterior tibial artery, 9. Dorsalis pedis artery

Page 91

Hit or miss

1. True, 2. False (the wall of a vein is thinner and more pliable), 3. False (veins contain valves), 4. True, 5. True, 6. False (it's about 5 L), 7. False (pulsations can only be felt where an artery lies near the skin), 8. True, 9. False (it occurs in capillaries), 10. True

Jumble gym

1. dorsalis pedis
2. ulnar
3. femoral
4. brachiocephalic
5. subclavian
6. transverse sinus
7. common iliac
8. aorta

Answer: Inferior vena cava

Page 92

A-maze-ing race

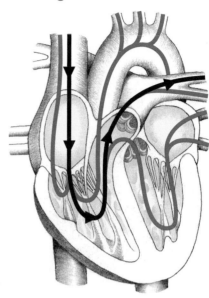

Answer: One of the branches of the left pulmonary artery; pathway of deoxygenated blood

Page 93

Team colors

1. Right jugular vein, 2. **Brachiocephalic artery**, 3. Pulmonary arteries, 4. Superior vena cava, 5. Inferior vena cava, 6. **Radial artery**, 7. **Ulnar artery**, 8. **Femoral artery**, 9. **Popliteal artery**, 10. **Temporal artery**, 11. **Right common carotid artery**, 12. Left subclavian artery, 13. Pulmonary veins, 14. Aorta, 15. Common iliac artery, 16. Common iliac vein, 17. **Posterior tibial artery**, 18. **Dorsalis pedis artery**

Page 94

Brain crunches

Commonly reported complaints: chest pain; irregular heartbeat or palpitations; shortness of breath on exertion, when lying down, or at night; cough; cyanosis or pallor; weakness; fatigue; unexplained weight change; swelling of the extremities; dizziness; headache; high or low blood pressure; peripheral skin changes (decreased hair distribution, skin color changes, or a thin, shiny appearance to skin); pain in extremities (leg pain or cramps)

Page 95

Gear up!

- ☑ Gloves
- ☐ Felt-tipped pen or marker
- ☐ Cotton-tipped applicators
- ☑ Stethoscope with bell and diaphragm
- ☑ Blood pressure cuff
- ☑ Measuring tape
- ☐ Ruler
- ☑ Povidone-iodine solution
- ☐ Penlight
- ☐ Otoscope
- ☐ Nasal speculum
- ☐ Tongue blade
- ☐ Tuning fork
- ☐ Syringes
- ☐ Needles
- ☐ Specimen containers

Photo finish

Anterior thorax view

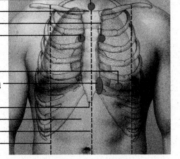

Sternoclavicular area
Suprasternal notch
Pulmonic area
Aortic area

Mitral (left ventricular) area
Tricuspid (right ventricular) area

Xiphoid process
Epigastric area
Midsternal line
Midclavicular line

Lateral thorax view

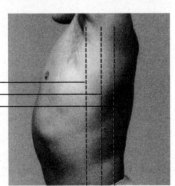

Anterior axillary line
Midaxillary line
Posterior axillary line

■ Page 96

Choose the best course

Assess general appearance (body shape and size), skin (color, temperature, turgor, and texture), and alertness.

▼

Inspect chest (note landmarks, pulsations, symmetry, retractions, heaves, and point of maximum impulse).

▼

Palpate precordium to find apical impulse, noting thrills; also palpate sternoclavicular, aortic, pulmonic, tricuspid, and epigastric areas for abnormal pulsations.

▼

Percuss heart to locate cardiac borders.

▼

Auscultate for heart sounds, murmurs, and friction rubs.

■ Page 97

Hit or miss

1. True, 2. False (they occur during both systole and diastole), 3. False (they're best heard with the patient sitting up and leaning forward), 4. True, 5. True, 6. False (this can be heard during inspiration), 7. True, 8. False (S_3 sounds are also common in young adults, especially in those with a high cardiac output, such as athletes), 9. True, 10. True

Match point

1. C, 2. E, 3. A, 4. F, 5. D, 6. B

■ Page 98

Step aerobics

1. **Forward-leaning position:** used to detect high-pitched sounds related to semilunar valve problems, such as pulmonic and aortic valve murmurs
2. **Left-lateral recumbent position:** used to detect low-pitched sounds, such as mitral valve murmurs and extra heart sounds

Team up!

Internal jugular vein
- Soft, undulating pulsation
- Pulsation detected about 1½″ (4 cm) above sternal notch
- Pulsation changes in response to position
- Pulsation changes in response to breathing
- Pulsation changes in response to palpation

Carotid artery
- No decrease noted when patient is upright
- No change noted when patient inhales
- Pulsation detected just lateral to trachea and below jaw line
- Brisk, localized pulsation
- No change noted with palpation

■ Page 99

You make the call

1. Popliteal pulse, 2. Carotid pulse, 3. Femoral pulse,
4. Dorsalis pedis pulse, 5. Radial pulse, 6. Brachial pulse,
7. Posterior tibial pulse

■ Page 100

Cross-training

Crossword answers:

Across: MURMURS, CHEST PAIN, HEART FAILURE, BRUIT, HYPOTENSION, TACHYCARDIA, AORTIC ANEURYSM, VENTRICULAR GALLOP, PALPITATION

Down: MYOCARDIAL, ARRHYTHMIA, CHESTERLIN (CHESTERION), ... AORTA, CYANOSIS, CARDIOGRAM, BRADYCARDIA, FATIGUE, EDEMA, DIION, VENA CAVA

■ Page 101

Strikeout

1. Sudden chest pain, lasting 30 minutes to 2 hours; shortness of breath; diaphoresis; weakness; anxiety; ~~hearing loss~~: <u>Acute myocardial infarction</u>
2. Moderate to severe bilateral leg edema, ~~visual halos~~, darkened skin, stasis ulcers around the ankles: <u>Venous insufficiency</u>
3. Paroxysmal or sustained palpitations; dizziness, weakness, and fatigue; ~~stomach pain~~; irregular, rapid, or slow pulse rate; decreased blood pressure; confusion: <u>Cardiac arrhythmias</u>
4. ~~Feeling of euphoria~~; aching, squeezing, heavy pressure; burning pain that usually subsides within 10 minutes: <u>Angina pectoris</u>
5. Sudden excruciating, tearing chest pain; pain radiating to back, neck, and shoulders; ~~Grade VI murmur~~; blood pressure difference between right and left arm: <u>Dissecting aortic aneurysm</u>

Mind sprints

Possible questions:

■ Can you describe the type of pain (dull, aching, stabbing, knifelike, sharp)?
■ Are you having the pain now?
■ Where do you feel the pain? Is it all in the same spot, or do you feel it radiating anywhere?
■ How long have you been having the pain? Is it a continuous pain, or does it come and go? If so, how long does it typically last?
■ Can you rate the pain on a scale of 0 to 10, with "0" being no pain and "10" being the worst pain you've ever experienced?
■ What were you doing when you first noticed the pain?
■ Do you have any other symptoms with the pain?
■ Does anything seem to aggravate the pain (stress, activities) or alleviate it?
■ Do you take any medication (prescribed or over-the-counter) to relieve the pain? Does it seem to help?
■ Were you ever previously treated for chest pain or diagnosed with a heart condition?

■ Page 102

In the ballpark

Edema grading scale

+1	Finger leaves slight imprint (2-mm indentation)
+2	4-mm indentation
+3	6-mm indentation
+4	Finger leaves deep imprint that only slowly returns to normal (8-mm indentation)

Pulses grading scale

4+	Bounding
3+	Increased
2+	Normal
1+	Weak
0	Absent

Winner's circle

1.

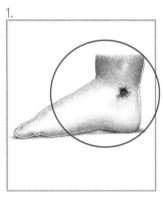
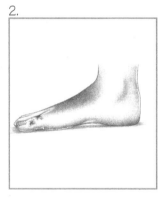

2.

■ Page 103

Match point

1. E, 2. G, 3. B, 4. C, 5. H, 6. A, 7. F, 8. D

■ Page 104

Train your brain

Answer: A forceful apical impulse can signal increased cardiac output.

Batter's box

1. left ventricle, 2. heart chamber, 3. valvular, 4. aortic, 5. aortic aneurysm; 6. thrill

■ Page 105

You make the call

1. Pulsus alternans, 2. Weak pulse, 3. Pulsus paradoxus, 4. Pulsus biferiens, 5. Bounding pulse, 6. Pulsus bigeminus

■ Page 106

Brain crunches

Factors affecting cardiovascular health
1. Stress, 2. Smoking, 3. Alcohol use, 4. Caffeine intake, 5. Exercise, 6. Dietary intake of fat and sodium, 7. Sedentary lifestyle or occupation

Criteria for describing murmurs
1. Quality (harsh, blowing, rumbling), 2. Timing (systole, diastole), 3. Intensity (loudness), 4. Location (heart chambers, valves), 5. Radiation (such as neck, axillae), 6. Pitch (high, medium, low)

Three-point conversion

1. Edema (swelling of the extremities), 2. Chest pain, 3. Dizziness (or vertigo)

Chapter 7

Page 111

Finish line

1. Oropharynx, 2. Thyroid cartilage, 3. Cricoid cartilage,
4. Mainstem bronchus, 5. Terminal bronchiole, 6. Alveolar duct,
7. Alveolar sac, 8. Nasopharynx, 9. Epiglottis,
10. Laryngopharynx, 11. Trachea, 12. Pleural space,
13. Respiratory bronchiole, 14. Alveolus

Page 112

Hit or miss

1. False (it's a flap of tissue that closes over the top of the larynx),
2. True, 3. True, 4. False (they're lined with parietal pleura),
5. True, 6. False (they contract with inhalation and relax with
exhalation), 7. True, 8. True

You make the call

1. Lung at rest: Inspiratory muscles are relaxed; atmospheric
   pressure is maintained in the tracheobronchial tree; no air
   movement occurs
2. Inhalation: Inspiratory muscles contract; diaphragm
   descends and flattens; negative alveolar pressure is
   maintained; air moves into lungs
3. Exhalation: Inspiratory muscles relax, causing lungs to recoil
   to resting size and position; diaphragm ascends, returning to
   resting position; positive alveolar pressure is maintained; air
   moves out of lungs

Page 113

Finish line

Anterior view
1. Suprasternal notch, 2. Manubrium, 3. Angle of Louis,
4. Right upper lobe, 5. Right middle lobe, 6. Right lower lobe,
7. Xiphoid process, 8. Clavicle, 9. First rib, 10. Left upper lobe,
11. Body of sternum, 12. Left lower lobe, 13. Midsternal line,
14. Right midclavicular line, 15. Right anterior axillary line

Posterior view
1. Spinous process of C7, 2. Left upper lobe, 3. Scapula,
4. Left lower lobe, 5. Vertebral line, 6. Left scapular line, 7. First
rib, 8. Right upper lobe, 9. Right middle lobe, 10. Right lower lobe

Page 114

Brain crunches

1. Dyspnea (shortness of breath), 2. Orthopnea (shortness of
breath while lying down), 3. Cough, 4. Sputum, 5. Wheezing,
6. Chest pain

Winner's circle

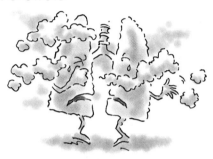

Answer: The patient should be instructed that second-hand
smoke poses many health risks and should be avoided whenever
possible.

Page 115

Mind sprints

Possible questions include:
■ Can you describe your cough to me?
■ Is the cough dry or productive?
■ What time of day do you cough most often, and when does this
occur (nighttime, morning, continuous)?
■ How long have you had the cough?
■ Have you noticed any changes in the cough recently? If so,
what?
■ Do you ever cough up blood or sputum? If so, how much (in
tsps, for example), how often, and what does it look like?
■ Do you have any other symptoms with the cough (wheezing,
pain)?
■ Does anything seem to make the cough better? Worse?
■ Are you taking any medication to control the cough?

Page 116

Match point

1. F, 2. B, 3. D, 4. G, 5. J, 6. A, 7. I, 8. H, 9. C, 10. E

■ Page 117

Step aerobics

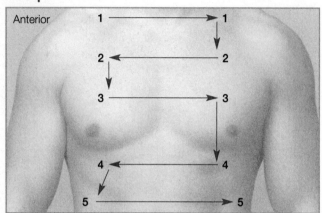

You make the call

Sound	Description	Clinical significance
Flat	Short, soft, high-pitched, extremely dull sound	Consolidation, as in atelectasis and extensive pleural effusion
Dull	**Medium intensity and pitch, moderate length, thudlike sound**	Solid area, as in lobar pneumonia
Resonant	Long, loud, low-pitched, hollow sound	**Normal lung tissue; bronchitis**
Hyperresonant	Very loud, lower-pitched sound	**Hyperinflated lung, as in emphysema or pneumothorax**
Tympanic	**Loud, high-pitched, moderate length, musical, drumlike sound**	Air collection, as in gastric bubbles or large pneumothorax

■ Page 118

Match point

1. C, 2. B, 3. D, 4. A

Photo finish

- Anterior thorax: 1. Bronchial, 2. Tracheal, 3. Bronchovesicular, 4. Vesicular
- Posterior thorax: 1. Tracheal, 2. Vesicular, 3. Bronchovesicular

■ Page 119

Team up!

One lung
- Pleural effusion
- Pneumothorax
- Tumor
- Mucus plugs in airways

Both lungs
- Atelectasis
- Severe bronchospasm
- Emphysema
- Shallow breathing

You make the call

1. Palpating for tactile fremitus: Checks for vibrations indicating tissue consolidation or obstructions
2. Chest percussion: Used to find boundaries of lungs, whether lungs are filled with air or fluid, and to evaluate the distance the diaphragm travels between inhalation and exhalation

■ Page 120

Choose the best course

| Ask patient to exhale. |

▼

| Percuss the back on one side to locate the upper edge of diaphragm. |

▼

| Use a pen to mark diaphragm's position at full expiration. |

▼

| Ask patient to inhale as deeply as possible. |

▼

| Percuss the back to locate diaphragm after patient breathes in fully. |

▼

| Use a pen to mark diaphragm's position at full inspiration. |

▼

| Repeat procedure on opposite side of back. |

▼

| Use a ruler or tape measure to determine distance between marks. |

Answer: The diaphragm normally moves 1¼″ to 2″ (3 to 5 cm) and should be equal on both the left and right sides.

■ Page 121

Three-point conversion

1. Whispered pectoriloquy: Numbers are almost indistinguishable over normal lung tissue; they're loud and clear over consolidated lung tissue.
2. Egophony: Letter "e" is muffled over normal lung tissue; over consolidated tissue, it sounds like the letter "a."
3. Bronchophony: Over normal lung tissue, the words "ninety-nine" are muffled; over consolidated tissue, they're unusually loud.

Strikeout

1. Tactile fremitus is decreased over areas where pleural fluid collects, at times when the patient speaks softly, ~~over large bronchial tubes~~, and in those with pneumothorax.
2. When palpating the chest wall, it should feel smooth, warm, ~~rigid~~, and dry.
3. Inspection of the skin, mouth, tongue, fingers, ~~toes~~, and nail beds may provide information about a patient's respiratory status.
4. Accessory inspiratory muscles include the trapezius, the sternocleidomastoid, ~~the diaphragm~~, and the scalenes.
5. Chest pain associated with a respiratory problem usually results from ~~asthma~~, pneumonia, pulmonary embolism, or pleural inflammation.

■ Page 122

Match point

1. D, 2. A, 3. C, 4. E, 5. F, 6. B

Train your brain

Answer: Patients with chest-wall deformities may more easily develop respiratory failure from a respiratory tract infection.

■ Page 123

Cross-training

Across and down crossword grid with answers:
- 1. PNEUMONIA (across), PNEUMOTHORAX (6 across)
- PULMONARY, CREPITUS, ASTHMA, RONCHI, TACHYPNEA
- SPUTUM (9 across), CRACKLES (10 across)
- DYSPNEA (11 across), CYANOSIS (12 across)
- WHEEZING, APNEA, CROUP

■ Page 124

Match point

1. B, 2. D, 3. A, 4. C

Hit or miss

1. True, 2. False (the patient may have completely normal lungs, but the lungs might be cramped within the chest), 3. True, 4. False (the diaphragm is flattened), 5. False (pectus carinatum is the other name for pigeon chest), 6. True

■ **Page 125**

In the ballpark

1. E, 2. C, 3. G, 4. A, 5. B, 6. D, 7. F

Brain crunches

1. Dyspnea, 2. Stridor, 3. Wheezing, 4. Decreased or absent breath sounds, 5. Use of accessory muscles, 6. Seesaw movement between chest and abdomen, 7. Inability to speak, 8. Cyanosis

■ **Page 126**

Jumble gym

1. **k u s s** m a u l
2. **b i o t**
3. b r a **d y** p n e a
4. **h** y p e r p n **e a**
5. t a **c** h y p n **e a**
6. a p n **e a**

Answer: Cheyne-Stokes

Team up!

Cough
- Atelectasis
- Lung cancer
- Pleural effusion

Dyspnea
- Acute respiratory distress syndrome
- Emphysema
- Pulmonary embolism

Hemoptysis
- Pneumonia
- Pulmonary edema
- Pulmonary tuberculosis

Wheezing
- Aspiration of a foreign body
- Asthma
- Chronic bronchitis

■ **Page 127**

You make the call

1. Hyperpnea, 2. Cheyne-Stokes respirations, 3. Bradypnea, 4. Biot's respirations, 5. Kussmaul's respirations, 6. Apnea, 7. Tachypnea

■ **Page 128**

Brain crunches

1. Crackles, 2. Wheezes, 3. Rhonchi, 4. Stridor, 5. Pleural friction rub

Hit or miss

1. False (they're heard during inhalation), 2. True, 3. True, 4. False ("death rattle" refers to coarse crackles), 5. False (they indicate an upper airway obstruction and require immediate attention)

■ Chapter 8

■ **Page 132**

Batter's box

1. mammary; 2. pectoralis major, serratus anterior, midaxillary; 3. nipple, areola; 4. Montgomery's tubercles, 5. glandular, fibrous, fatty; 6. lactiferous; 7. lymph; 8. breast cancer; 9. puberty, asymmetrically; 10. menstrual cycle; 11. corpus luteum, placenta, 12. estrogen

■ **Page 133**

Finish line

1. Collecting and main duct, 2. Fibrous septa, 3. Glandular lobe, 4. Acini of lobe, 5. Areola, 6. Montgomery's tubercle, 7. Nipple, 8. Lactiferous duct orifice, 9. Lactiferous duct

Hit or miss

1. True, 2. False (they attach to the chest wall musculature), 3. True, 4. False (the pectoral nodes drain lymph from the anterior chest; the subscapular nodes drain the posterior chest and part of the arm), 5. False (the opposite is true), 6. False (pigmentation varies among races, getting darker as skin tone darkens)

■ Page 134

Finish line

1. Supraclavicular, 2. Infraclavicular, 3. Brachial (lateral), 4. Midaxillary (central), 5. Internal mammary, 6. Pectoral (anterior), 7. Subscapular (posterior)

Brain crunches

1. Breast pain, 2. Nipple discharge or rash, 3. Lumps or masses, 4. Other changes (such as skin dimpling, nipple retraction, and skin or vein changes)

■ Page 135

Strikeout

1. Breast skin should be smooth, undimpled, ~~very warm~~, and the same color as the rest of the skin.
2. Breasts are commonly examined with the patient lying supine with her hand behind her head on the side you're examining, sitting with arms at her sides, holding her arms over her head, ~~lying on her stomach with arms extended to the side~~, and standing with her hands on the back of a chair while leaning forward.
3. Nipples should be examined for size and shape, discharge, elasticity, ~~reflexes~~, and protrusion.
4. Nodularity, ~~irregular shape~~, fullness, and mild tenderness of breasts are common premenstrual symptoms that may be noted during a breast exam.
5. Palpation typically includes gently rotating three fingers in concentric circles against the chest wall, ~~moving from the chest periphery toward the nipple~~, including the tail of Spence, and gently squeezing the areola and nipple with a gloved hand.
6. Palpable lymph nodes typically are ~~hard~~, small, and nontender.

You make the call

1. After pregnancy, 2. During adulthood (having never given birth), 3. Between ages 10 and 14, 4. During pregnancy, 5. Before age 8, 6. After menopause

■ Page 136

Team colors

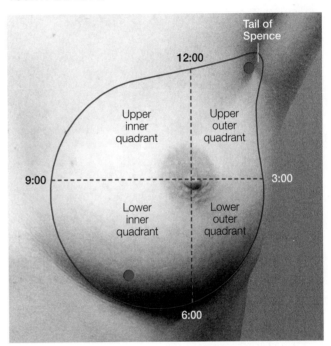

Brain crunches

1. Size (in centimeters), 2. Shape (round, discoid, regular, or irregular), 3. Consistency (soft, firm, or hard), 4. Mobility, 5. Degree of tenderness, 6. Location (using quadrant or clock method)

■ Page 137

You make the call

1. Dimpling, 2. Peau d'orange

Team up!

Benign lesion
- Round and lobular
- Well demarcated; feels firm to soft
- Very mobile; feels slippery
- Nontender; no skin retraction

Malignant lesion
- Irregular or star-shaped
- Poorly defined edges; feels firm to hard
- Fixed and single
- Usually nontender with skin retraction

■ Page 138
Match point
1. F, 2. C, 3. B, 4. G, 5. E, 6. H, 7. A, 8. D

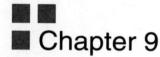

■ Chapter 9

■ Page 142
Batter's box
1. mouth, 2. anus, 3. peristalsis, 4. esophagus, 5. intestines, 6. chyme, 7. carbohydrates, 8. colon, 9. feces, 10. liver, 11. bile, 12. gallbladder, 13. pancreas

■ Page 143
Jumble gym
1. h e a r t **b** u r n
2. **r** e c t a l **b** l e e d i n g
3. n a u s e a
4. f l a t u l e n c e
5. v o **m** i t i n **g**
6. d i a r **r** h e a
7. d **y** s p h a g i a
8. c o **n** s t i p a t i o n
9. s t o **m** a c h a c h e

Answer: Borborygmus

Mind sprints
Possible questions:
■ How would you describe your diarrhea (color, amount, consistency)?
■ How often does it occur?
■ Is it a new or recurring problem?
■ When did you first notice it?
■ Have you noticed any other changes in your bowel patterns, such as constipation or flatus?
■ Do you ever see any blood in your stool?
■ Are you experiencing any other GI-related problems (belching, nausea, vomiting, stomachaches)?
■ Are you taking anything to treat the diarrhea?
■ What medications do you regularly take? Have you recently started taking any new prescriptions?
■ Have you recently traveled abroad?
■ Does anyone in your family have a GI disorder?
■ Do you use alcohol, caffeine, or tobacco?

■ Page 144
Finish line
1. Mouth, 2. Liver, 3. Gallbladder, 4. Duodenum, 5. Ascending colon, 6. Cecum, 7. Vermiform appendix, 8. Epiglottis, 9. Pharynx, 10. Esophagus, 11. Stomach, 12. Pancreas, 13. Transverse colon, 14. Descending colon, 15. Jejunum, 16. Ileum, 17. Sigmoid colon, 18. Rectum

■ Page 145
Brain crunches
1. Ulcerative colitis, 2. Colorectal cancer, 3. Peptic ulcers, 4. Gastric cancer, 5. Diabetes, 6. Alcoholism, 7. Crohn's disease

Strikeout
1. Have you ever been diagnosed with a GI illness, such as an ulcer, inflammatory bowel disease, ~~von Willebrand's disease~~, irritable bowel syndrome, or gastroesophageal reflux?
2. Are you currently taking any ~~multivitamins~~, aspirin, nonsteroidal anti-inflammatory drugs, antibiotics, or opioid analgesics?
3. Have you noticed any changes in appetite, ability to chew or swallow, bowel habits, or ~~resistance to disease~~?
4. What's your usual diet, exercise routine, ~~sexual pattern~~, sleep pattern, and oral hygiene?
5. Do you have any allergies to ~~pets~~, foods, or medicines?
6. Have you noticed any changes in the color, odor, ~~temperature~~, amount, or appearance of your stool?

■ Page 146
Batter's box
1. mouth, abdomen, rectum; 2. auscultation, percussion, palpation; 3. inspection; 4. quadrants; 5. umbilicus, costal margins; 6. navel, symphysis pubis; 7. normal, hyperactive, hypoactive; 8. before mealtimes; 9. air, fluid; 10. clockwise

■ Page 147

Match point

1. D, 2. A, 3. B, 4. C

You make the call

Right upper quadrant
- Right lobe of liver
- Gallbladder
- Pylorus
- Duodenum
- Head of the pancreas
- Hepatic flexure of the colon
- Portions of the ascending and transverse colon

Left upper quadrant
- Left lobe of the liver
- Stomach
- Body of the pancreas
- Splenic flexure of the colon
- Portions of the transverse and descending colon

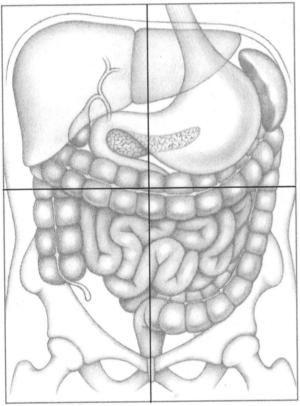

Right lower quadrant
- Cecum and appendix
- Portion of the ascending colon

Left lower quadrant
- Sigmoid colon
- Portion of the descending colon

■ Page 148

Gear up!

- ☑ Stethoscope
- ☑ Gloves
- ☐ Cotton-tipped applicators
- ☑ Lubricant
- ☐ Otoscope
- ☑ Ruler (in centimeters)
- ☑ Flexible tape measure
- ☐ Blood pressure cuff
- ☐ Snellen chart
- ☐ Urine specimen container
- ☑ Guaiac test kit
- ☐ Forceps
- ☐ Syringe
- ☑ Pen
- ☐ Scale
- ☑ Tongue blade
- ☐ Thermometer
- ☐ Mirror
- ☐ Tuning fork
- ☐ Safety pin
- ☑ Penlight
- ☐ Speculum
- ☑ Drape
- ☑ Small pillow
- ☑ Percussion hammer

Match point

1. C, 2. E, 3. F, 4. A, 5. B, 6. D

■ Page 149

Team up!

Hyperactive bowel sounds
- Diarrhea
- Laxative use
- Constipation

Hypoactive bowel sounds
- Use of opioid analgesics
- Peritonitis
- Ileus
- Bowel obstruction or torsion

You make the call

1. Right renal artery, 2. Aorta, 3. Right iliac artery, 4. Right femoral artery, 5. Left renal artery, 6. Left iliac artery, 7. Left femoral artery

■ Page 150

You make the call

1. Dullness: Heard over solid organs, such as the liver, kidney, or feces-filled intestines
2. Tympany: Heard over hollow organs, such as an empty stomach or bowel, where air is normally present

Step aerobics

Assessment: Measuring the liver
Procedure steps
1. Percuss to identify upper border of liver dullness. Start in right midclavicular line in an area of lung resonance, and percuss downward toward the liver. Mark the spot where the sound changes to dullness.
2. Starting in the right midclavicular line at a level below the umbilicus, lightly percuss upward toward the liver. Mark the spot where the sound changes from tympany to dullness.
3. Measure the vertical span between the two marked spots.

■ Page 151

Hit or miss

1. True, 2. True, 3. False (auscultate for vascular sounds with the bell of the stethoscope), 4. True, 5. False (they should be palpated last), 6. False (light palpation is used for these reasons), 7. True, 8. False (for deep palpation, depress 2″ to 3″ (5 to 7.5 cm), 9. False (never palpate a rigid abdomen; this could cause pain or rupture an inflamed organ), 10. False (percussion is used for this reason)

■ Page 152

Cross-training

										C	O	L	O	N
				S	T	R	I	A	E		C			
				A					C		U			
				L			E		U		M			
		A	S	C	I	T	E	S	M					P
				V			O							E
				A			P		H					R
		U					H		Y					I
		M					A		P		S			
		B		E	P	I	G	L	O	T	T	I	S	
		I			A	U		A		O			T	
S	P	L	E	E	N		S		C		M		A	
		I			C				T		A		L	
		C			R				I		C		S	
		A			E				V		H		I	
		L	A	X	A	T	I	V	E	S			S	
					S									

■ Page 153

You make the call

1. Standard palpation of liver
2. Hooking the liver

Match point

1. D, 2. C, 3. A, 4. E, 5. F, 6. B

■ Page 154

You make the call

Palpating the spleen: Stand on the patient's right side. Use your left hand to support his posterior left lower rib cage, and ask him to take a deep breath. Then, with your right hand on his abdomen, press up and in toward the spleen.

■ Page 155

Train your brain

Answer: A bulging abdomen may indicate bladder distention or hernia.

You make the call

Assessing for ascites: Have an assistant place the ulnar edge of her hand firmly on the patient's abdomen at its midline. Then stand facing the patient's head, and place your right hand against the patient's left flank. Give the right abdomen a firm tap with your left hand and observe and feel for a "fluid wave" ripple across the abdomen.

■ Page 156

Choose the best course

Inspect the perianal area.

▼

Put on gloves.

▼

Spread buttocks to expose anus and surrounding tissue, and check for abnormalities.

▼

Ask patient to strain as if having a bowel movement.

▼

After applying water-soluble lubricant to index finger, insert finger, aiming toward umbilicus.

▼

Palpate rectum in a clockwise, then a counterclockwise direction.

▼

Inspect glove for stool, blood, and mucus and test fecal matter with a guaiac test.

■ Page 157

Brain crunches

1. Internal fissures, 2. External fissures, 3. Lesions, 4. Scars, 5. Inflammation, 6. Discharge, 7. Rectal prolapse, 8. External hemorrhoids, 9. Internal hemorrhoids, 10. Polyps

Match point

1. C, 2. B, 3. A, 4. D

■ Page 158

Batter's box

1. pneumonia, 2. lactose intolerance, 3. Turner's, 4. duodenal, 5. hematochezia, 6. constipation, 7. Cullen's, 8. umbilical hernia, 9. bowel obstruction, 10. peritoneal, 11. liver

■ Page 159

Strikeout

1. During palpation of the rectum, the rectal walls should normally feel soft and smooth, ~~mucous or bloody~~, and without masses or fecal impaction.
2. Dysphagia can be caused by an obstruction, achalasia of the lower esophagogastric junction, stroke, Parkinson's disease, or ~~dysmenorrhea~~.
3. Ascites can be caused by ~~thyrotoxicosis~~, advanced liver disease, heart failure, pancreatitis, or cancer.
4. Hyperactive bowel sounds unrelated to hunger may be caused by diarrhea, laxative use, early bowel obstruction, or ~~paralytic ileus~~.

■ Page 160

Match point

1. E, 2. G, 3. C, 4. F, 5. A, 6. I, 7. D, 8. B, 9. H

Chapter 10

■ Page 164

Hit or miss

1. False (the vagina is part of the reproductive system, not the urinary system), 2. True, 3. False (they're located on either side of the lumbar vertebrae), 4. True, 5. True, 6. True, 7. False (the fundus is the upper portion of the uterus; the cervix protrudes into the vagina), 8. False (the ovaries release estrogen and progesterone), 9. True, 10. False (fertilization usually occurs in the fallopian tubes)

■ Page 165

Finish line

1. Renal vein, 2. Inferior vena cava, 3. Ureters, 4. Bladder, 5. Renal artery, 6. Kidneys, 7. Abdominal aorta, 8. Urethra

In the ballpark

1. F, 2. A, 3. E, 4. G, 5. B, 6. C, 7. D

■ Page 166

Finish line

External genitalia
1. Prepuce of clitoris, 2. Labia majora, 3. Labia minora, 4. Bartholin's glands, 5. Mons pubis, 6. Skene's glands, 7. Urethral orifice, 8. Vaginal introitus, 9. Perineum

Internal genitalia
1. Uterine fundus, 2. Fallopian tube, 3. Ovary, 4. Uterine cavity, 5. External fornix, 6. Cervix, 7. Vaginal vault

■ Page 167

Brain crunches

1. Output changes (such as polyuria, oliguria, anuria)
2. Voiding pattern changes (such as hesitancy, frequency, urgency, nocturia, incontinence)
3. Urine color changes
4. Pain

Jumble gym

1. kidney stones
2. hypertension
3. diabetes
4. allergic reactions
5. urinary tract infections
6. cardiovascular disease
7. nephrotoxic drugs

Answer: Urinary tract health

■ Page 168

Brain crunches

1. Pain
2. Vaginal discharge
3. Abnormal uterine bleeding
4. Pruritus
5. Infertility

Mind sprints

Possible questions:
■ How old were you when you first began to menstruate?
■ How long do your menses typically last?
■ How often do you menstruate (every 28 days, more or less frequently)?
■ Do you experience cramps, spotting, or unusually heavy or light flow with your menses?
■ Do you have spotting between menses?
■ Do you have any other symptoms or problems (pain, itching, unusual discharge, or odors)?
■ Are you sexually active? If so, can you describe your sexual practices and number of partners? Do you ever experience pain with intercourse? Do you use birth control? If so, what kind?
■ Have you ever been pregnant? If so, can you give specifics (number of pregnancies, births, miscarriages or abortions, types of deliveries [vaginal or cesarean], complications)?
■ Have you ever had a sexually transmitted disease or been tested for HIV? If you have been tested for HIV, was the result positive or negative?
■ When was your last Pap test, and what was the result?

■ Page 169

Gear up!

☑ Gloves
☐ Penlight
☐ Percussion hammer
☑ Blood pressure cuff
☑ Vaginal speculum
☑ Water-soluble lubricant
☐ Specimen containers
☐ Cotton-tipped applicators
☐ Tongue blade
☐ Tuning fork
☑ Scale
☐ Body mass index chart
☐ Otoscope
☐ Guaiac test kit
☐ Ophthalmoscope
☐ Dextrostix kit
☑ Gown and drape
☐ 20-gauge needle
☐ Syringes
☐ Tape measure
☐ Povidone-iodine solution
☑ Warm water

Train your brain

Answer: Checking your patient's vital signs, weight, and mental status can provide clues about renal dysfunction.

■ Page 170

Strikeout

1. Normally, the skin over the kidney and bladder areas should be free from lesions, ~~hair follicles~~, discoloration, inflammation, and swelling.
2. Normal external genital discharge may be clear and stretchy, white and opaque, or ~~yellow and curdlike~~ depending on the time of the patient's menstrual cycle.
3. You should notify the practitioner and obtain a specimen if the patient's vestibule (especially around the Skene's and Bartholin's glands) shows any signs of swelling, ~~pinkness~~, lesions, discharge, or unusual odor.
4. Inspection of the patient's ~~umbilicus~~, external genitalia, and pubic hair can help to assess her sexual maturity.
5. It's possible to milk and culture discharge from the patient's urethra, ~~clitoris~~, Skene's glands, and Bartholin's glands when these areas are swollen, inflamed, or tender.
6. Common types of specula used to inspect internal genitalia include Pederson, Graves', plastic, and ~~Nagashima Takahashi~~ varieties.
7. The cervix is commonly examined for color, position, ~~temperature~~, shape and size, mucosal integrity, and discharge.
8. Pain noted while palpating the patient's cervical area may be an indication of inflammation of the uterus, ovaries, fallopian tubes, ligaments of the uterus, or ~~inferior vena cava~~.
9. Rectovaginal palpation helps to assess the rectum, the posterior part of the uterus, ~~the ovaries~~, and the pelvic cavity.
10. A bimanual examination is used to palpate the uterus, ovaries, and ~~mons pubis~~.

■ Page 171

You make the call

Assessment procedure: Inserting a speculum

1. **Initial insertion:** Insert index and middle fingers of nondominant hand about 1″ (2.5 cm) into vagina, and spread them open to exert pressure on posterior portion. Hold speculum in dominant hand, and insert blades.
2. **Deeper insertion:** As patient bears down, point speculum slightly downward and insert blades until base touches your fingers still in vagina.
3. **Rotate and open:** Rotate speculum in same plane as vagina, and withdraw your fingers. Open blades as far as possible and lock them.

Hit or miss

1. True, 2. False (only warm water should be used; anything else may be bacteriostatic and can alter Pap test results), 3. True, 4. True

■ Page 172

You make the call

1. **Nulliparous os:** the os of a woman who has never given birth vaginally
2. **Parous os:** the os of a woman who has given birth vaginally

Match point

1. B, 2. C, 3. A

■ Page 173

Cross-training

Across answers: 1. AMENORRHEA, 3. DYSURIA, 6. RECTOCELE, 7. GENITALWARTS, 9. DYSMENORRHEA, 12. CANDIDIASIS, 13. HEMATURIA, 14. NOCTURIA, 15. POLYURIA, 16. PMS, 17. VAGINITIS

```
A M E N O R R H E A     D Y S U R I A
        N                         N
        D                   C     C
      R E C T O C E L E     H     O
        M                   L     N
          G E N I T A L W A R T S
    C       T                 M   I
  D Y S M E N O R R H E A     Y   N
    S       I                 D   E
    T       O   U   H         I   N
    O       S   T   E         A   N
    C     C A N D I D I A S I S   C
    E     Y     S   I
    L     S         T
  H E M A T U R I A           A
        I                     N
  N O C T U R I A             C
        I           P O L Y U R I A
    P M S
              V A G I N I T I S
```

■ Page 174

Match point

1. D, 2. A, 3. B, 4. E, 5. C

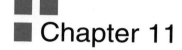

Chapter 11

■ Page 178

Hit or miss

1. True, 2. False (testosterone is produced by the testes in the reproductive system as well as by the adrenal glands), 3. True, 4. False (this is the penis), 5. False (semen and sperm are ejaculated), 6. True, 7. False (this is the epididymis), 8. True, 9. True, 10. True, 11. True, 12. False (it's longer in order to pass through the erectile tissue of the penis), 13. True, 14. False (the left side is typically longer because the left spermatic cord is longer), 15. False (these are primary characteristics; secondary include appearance of facial and body hair, muscle development, and voice changes)

■ Page 179

Finish line

1. Symphysis pubis, 2. Prostate gland, 3. Vas deferens, 4. Corpus cavernosum, 5. Urethra, 6. Penis, 7. Glans penis, 8. Corona, 9. Prepuce (foreskin), 10. Urethral meatus, 11. Bladder, 12. Seminal vesicle, 13. Common ejaculatory duct, 14. Epididymis, 15. Testicle, 16. Scrotum

Brain crunches

1. Penile discharge
2. Erectile dysfunction
3. Infertility
4. Scrotal or inguinal masses, pain, or tenderness

■ Page 180

Strikeout

1. Sores, lumps, ulcers, or ~~absence of hair~~ on the penis can signal a sexually transmitted disease.
2. During the health assessment, it's important to ask about the patient's history of diabetes, kidney stones, bladder infections, ~~hypotension,~~ and catheterization.
3. Scrotal swelling can be a sign of ~~hiatal hernia,~~ inguinal hernia, hematocele, epididymitis, or testicular cancer.
4. To assess sexual risk-taking behaviors, it's appropriate to ask about a patient's sexual preference, ~~circumcision status,~~ usual sexual practices, HIV status, and birth control measures.
5. Factors that can raise the scrotal temperature and temporarily diminish a patient's sperm include frequent bicycle or motorcycle riding, taking hot baths, using an athletic supporter, and ~~wearing boxer shorts~~.

Match point

1. C, 2. F, 3. A, 4. G, 5. D, 6. B, 7. E

■ Page 181

You make the call

1. **Palpating for an indirect inguinal hernia:** Place gloved finger on the neck of the scrotum, and insert it into the inguinal canal. Ask patient to bear down. A hernia will feel like a soft mass at your fingertip.
2. **Palpating the prostate gland:** Insert a lubricated gloved finger into the rectum, and palpate the anterior rectal wall, just past the anorectal ring.

■ Page 182

Cross-training

			¹N		²P			³V				
			E		R			A				
⁴P	A	R	A	P	H	I	M	O	S	I	S	
			H		A			D			⁵S	
	⁶P		R		P		⁷J	E			E	
⁸H	R		O		I		O	F			B	
E	O		T		S		C	E			A	
M	S		I		M		K	R			C	
A	T		C				I	E			E	
⁹T	R	A	N	S	I	L	L	U	M	I	N	A	T	I	O	N
U	T		Y				S	C			U	
R	E		N		¹⁰H			H			S	
I			D		E						C	
A		¹¹U	R	E	M	I	C	F	R	O	S	T	Y
		O			N						S	
¹²S	M	E	G	M	A			I			T	
		E						A			S	

■ Page 183

Match point

1. B, 2. D, 3. A, 4. C

Jumble gym

1. erectile dysfunction
2. hydrocele
3. benign prostatic hyperplasia
4. hypospadias
5. epispadias
6. testicular tumor

Answer: Infertility

■ Page 184

Hit or miss

1. True, 2. True, 3. False (both conditions are congenital), 4. False (these are signs and symptoms of gonococcal urethritis), 5. True

Team colors

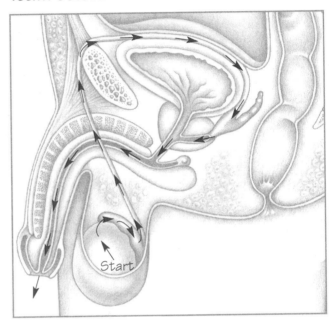

Start

Chapter 12

Page 188

Batter's box

1. 206, 2. organs, 3. tissues, 4. bone marrow, 5. joints, 6. movement, 7. nonsynovial, 8. synovial; 9. ligaments, 10. ball-and-socket, 11. hinge; 12. contractile; 13. tendons; 14. bursae; 15. cartilage; 16. synovial fluid

Page 189

Team up!

Axial skeleton
- Hyoid
- Sternum
- Skull
- Ribs
- Facial bones
- Vertebrae

Appendicular skeleton
- Shoulders
- Legs
- Pelvis
- Arms

Finish line

1. Joint capsule, 2. Synovial fluid, 3. Cartilage, 4. Bone

Page 190

Finish line

Anterior view
1. Maxilla, 2. Mandible, 3. Clavicle, 4. Sternum, 5. Humerus, 6. Iliac crest, 7. Ulna, 8. Radius, 9. Greater trochanter, 10. Acetabulum, 11. Femur, 12. Patella, 13. Tarsal, 14. Metatarsals, 15. Phalanges, 16. Carpal, 17. Metacarpals, 18. Phalanges

Posterior view
1. Cervical vertebrae, 2. Acromion process, 3. Scapula, 4. Thoracic vertebrae, 5. Rib, 6. Lumbar vertebrae, 7. Ilium, 8. Sacrum, 9. Coccyx, 10. Ischium, 11. Tibia, 12. Fibula

Page 191

Match point

1. G, 2. L, 3. C, 4. B, 5. K, 6. D, 7. F, 8. H, 9. A, 10. J, 11. I, 12. E

Page 192

Jumble gym

1. pain
2. swelling
3. stiffness
4. deformity
5. weakness
6. achiness
7. fracture

Answer: Emergencies

Brain crunches

1. Signs and symptoms (pain, weakness, edema, deformities, grating sounds)
2. History of gout, arthritis, tuberculosis, cancer, or osteoporosis
3. Recent blunt or penetrating trauma (car accident, fall)
4. Current range of motion
5. Use or heat, cold, or assistive devices (cane, walker, brace)
6. Medications taken regularly (corticosteroids, potassium-depleting diuretics)
7. Lifestyle (job, hobbies, activities of daily living, exercise)

Page 193

Hit or miss

1. False (the CNS and musculoskeletal system are interrelated and should be assessed together), 2. False (inspection and palpation are used for this assessment), 3. True, 4. False (they don't require any effort), 5. True, 6. False (it's an indicator of muscular dystrophy)

You make the call

Gowers' sign: A positive Gowers' sign (an inability to lift the trunk from a supine position without using the hands and arms to brace and push) indicates pelvic muscle weakness, as occurs in muscular dystrophy and spinal muscle atrophy.

■ Page 194

In the ballpark

Neck: 40° touching ear to shoulder; 45° forward flexion; 55° backward extension
Shoulder: 180° flexion; 45° extension (normal range is 30° to 50°)
Wrist: 55° lateral rotation; 20° medial rotation
Hip: 45° abduction; 30° adduction
Knee: 125° flexion (normal range is 120° to 130°); 0° extension (normal range is 0° to 15°)
Foot: 45° plantar flexion; 20° dorsiflexion

■ Page 195

Batter's box

1. temporomandibular joint, 2. kyphosis, 3. lordosis; 4. spine, 5. rheumatoid arthritis, 6. %

Winner's circle

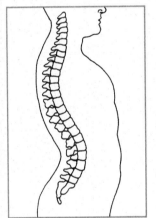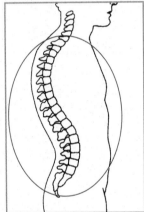

■ Page 196

You make the call

1. **Tinel's sign:** Light percussion of the transverse carpal tunnel ligament over the median nerve can produce discomfort (numbness, tingling shooting into the palm and fingers)—a sign of carpal tunnel syndrome.
2. **Phalen's maneuver:** Flexing the wrist for 30 seconds can cause pain or numbness in the hand or fingers—also a sign of carpal tunnel syndrome.

Brain crunches

1. Fractures
2. Dislocations
3. Amputations
4. Crush injuries
5. Serious lacerations

■ Page 197

You make the call

Bulge sign: Indicates excess fluid in the joint

Steps
1. Give two to four firm strokes to the medial side of the knee to displace excess fluid.
2. Tap the lateral aspect of the knee while checking for a fluid wave on the medial aspect.

■ Page 198

Jumble gym

1. spasms
2. tics
3. contractures
4. tremors
5. hypertrophy
6. fasciculations

Answer: Muscles

You make the call

1. Heberden's node
2. Bouchard's node

Clinical significance: Usually hard and painless, these bony and cartilaginous enlargements typically occur in middle-aged and elderly patients with osteoarthritis.

■ *Page 199*

Match point

1. B, 2. D, 3. F, 4. A, 5. C, 6. E

You make the call

1. Ankle strength: Plantar flexion
2. Triceps strength
3. Biceps strength
4. Ankle strength: Dorsiflexion

■ *Page 200*

Cross-training

				¹S	P	A	S	²M	S				
								U			³B		
⁴T	E	N	D	O	N	I	T	I	S		O		
M							⁵K				W		
J		⁶C	A	R	P	A	L	T	U	N	N	E	L
							L		O				E
							A		C				G
							R		K				G
⁷D	I	S	L	O	C	A	T	E	D		K		E
							Y		N		D		
	⁸S	⁹C	O	L	I	O	S	I	S		E		
¹⁰L		R						T	E		¹¹B		
O		E		¹²A				R	D		U		
R		P		T				O			N		
D		I		R		¹³K	Y	P	H	O	S	I	S
¹⁴F	O	O	T	D	R	O	P		H		O		
S		U		P				Y			N		
I		S		H									
S				Y									

■ *Page 201*

Train your brain

Answer: Ball-and-socket joints allow the shoulders and hips to move freely.

Brain crunches

Possible problems:
- Deformities
- Edema
- Nodules
- Calluses
- Bunions
- Corns
- Ingrown toenails
- Plantar warts
- Trophic ulcers

■ *Page 202*

Strike out

1. Painful and audible knee pops, inability to extend the leg fully, pronounced crepitus, ~~a negative bulge sign~~, and sudden buckling are all considered abnormal.
2. Referred shoulder pain may be due to a ~~dislocation~~, heart attack, or ruptured ectopic pregnancy.
3. Examples of spinal deformities include scoliosis, ~~ecchymosis~~, kyphosis, and lordosis.
4. Temporomandibular joint dysfunction can lead to local swelling, crepitus, pain, ~~sciatica~~, and lockjaw.
5. Hands should be carefully inspected for tenderness, ~~maxillary edema~~, nodules, webbing between fingers, and boggy joints.
6. Corticosteroids can cause ~~swelling~~, muscle weakness, myopathy, osteoporosis, pathologic fractures, and avascular necrosis of the heads of the femur and humerus.
7. Osteoporosis causes a decrease in bone mass that leaves bones porous, ~~calcified~~, brittle, and prone to fracture.
8. Knitting, playing football or tennis, ~~swimming~~, working at a computer, and doing construction work can cause repetitive stress injuries.
9. Muscle atrophy may result from neuromuscular disease or injury, metabolic and endocrine disorders, ~~extensive exercising~~, prolonged immobility, or aging.
10. Muscle spasms commonly result from muscle fatigue, exercise, electrolyte imbalances, ~~use of potassium-sparing diuretics~~, and pregnancy.

■ Page 203

Team up!

Upper extremities
- Acromion process
- Carpal
- Humerus
- Metacarpal
- Phalanges
- Radius
- Ulna

Lower extremities
- Acetabulum
- Femur
- Fibula
- Greater trochanter
- Metatarsals
- Patella
- Phalanges
- Tarsal
- Tibia

Torso
- Cervical vertebrae
- Clavicle
- Coccyx
- Iliac crest
- Ilium
- Ischium
- Lumbar vertebrae
- Rib
- Scapula
- Sternum
- Thoracic vertebrae

■ Page 204

Match point

1. F, 2. A, 3. D, 4. B, 5. G, 6. C, 7. E

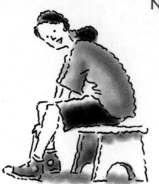

Notes

Notes

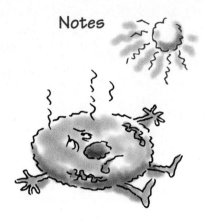

Notes

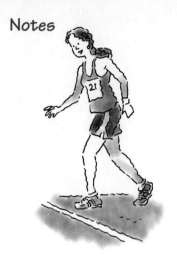

Notes

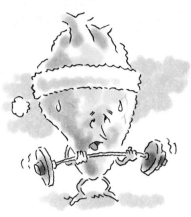

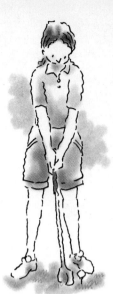

Notes

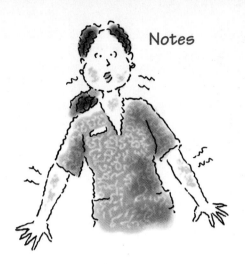

Notes

Notes

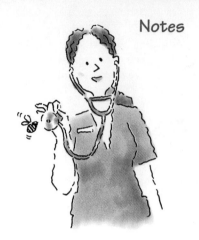

Notes

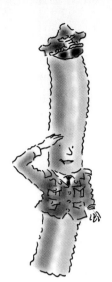

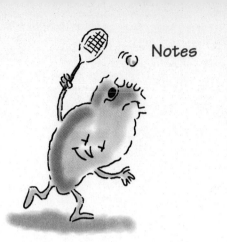

Notes

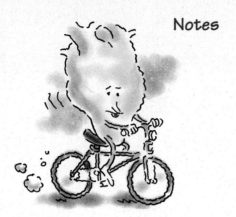

Notes

Notes

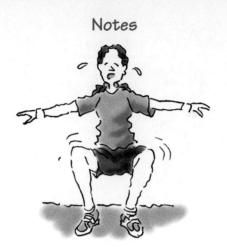